REIKI ILLUSTRATED

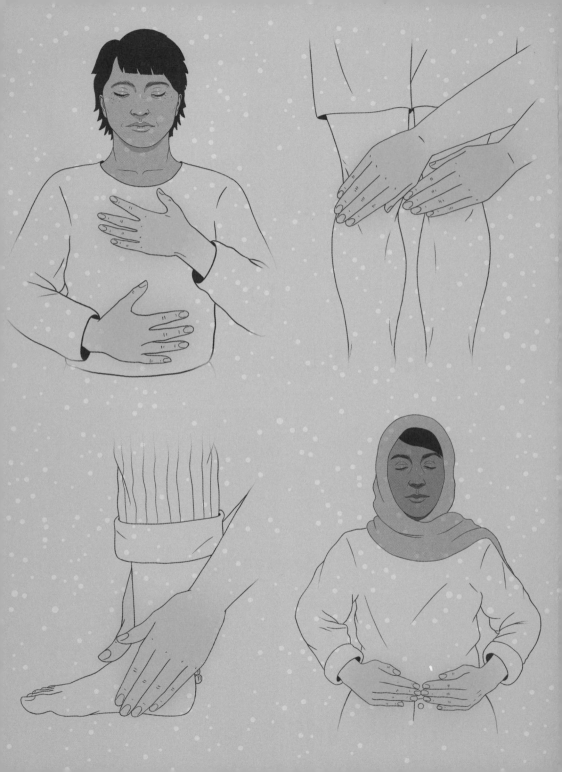

Reiki
ILLUSTRATED

THE VISUAL REFERENCE GUIDE
of Hand Positions, Symbols,
and Treatment Sequences
for Common Conditions

Hae Lee

ZEITGEIST · NEW YORK

Published in the United States by Zeitgeist, an imprint of Zeitgeist™, a division of Penguin Random House LLC, New York.
zeitgeistpublishing.com

Zeitgeist™ is a trademark of Penguin Random House LLC

ISBN: 9780593435656
Ebook ISBN: 9780593435762

Illustrations by Natalie Foss
Author photograph © Shyanne Pozon
Illustrator photograph © Rob Williamson
Book design by Katy Brown and Emma Hall

Printed in the United States of America
2nd Printing

Contents

Introduction

In 1922, a Japanese Buddhist monk named Mikao Usui went on a spiritual quest on Mount Kurama in Japan, during which he achieved enlightenment. After fasting and meditating for 21 days, Usui was bestowed the revelation that he could channel healing energy through his hands. His experience helped him develop the system of healing that we now call Reiki. According to the inscription on his memorial tomb and various sources, Usui trained about 2,000 students.

After graduating from college, I spent a lot of time in solitude, wondering about my life purpose, and I came to realize that my gift has always been and will always be helping people heal. I remember asking the universe for guidance, and countless synchronicities and signs led me to Reiki, an energy healing modality that I barely knew anything about. There was an indescribable voice in my head that instructed me to lead with my curiosity and become certified in Reiki. By following one breadcrumb after another from the universe, I birthed a Reiki-based healing practice called STAY+VIBE. Looking back, I am so grateful I listened to my inner calling at such a young age, because sharing and teaching this healing modality has been one of the most rewarding experiences in my life, and I wouldn't trade it for anything.

Maybe you can relate; perhaps Reiki somehow miraculously called and found you too. I believe that universal intelligence is always conspiring to answer our questions, but it is our job to look deep and inward so that we can find and honor our inner voice.

I applaud you for leading with your intuition, curiosity, open heart, and mind—which is what's brought you here. My hope is that you use this book to refresh your knowledge, supplement your training materials, and strengthen your confidence and connection to this healing modality.

This book follows the Usui Shiki Ryoho/Holy Fire® III system of healing and teachings of William Lee Rand, the founder of the International Center for Reiki Training (ICRT), from whom I had the pleasure of receiving placements and training.

PART I

Hand Positions & Symbols

This part of the book covers basic key concepts and best practices to remember when channeling Reiki, whether you are practicing on yourself or others, in person or from a distance. A list of standard hand positions is included to use as a guide when you are not sure where to place your hands, as well as the Reiki symbols to help you better connect with the universal life force energy and enhance your healing experience. I hope this serves you!

CHAPTER ONE

Key Concepts and Practices

In this chapter, I review the background information and core key concepts—the Reiki principles, the three pillars, and the energy body as it pertains to Reiki. I also include helpful techniques, sequencing, and tips to remember when holding both in-person and distant treatments. I include specific steps on how I carry out my treatments from beginning to end to demonstrate what has worked for me and my clients over the years.

Reiki Principles

Reiki is not only a healing modality but also an integral part of personal development and spiritual growth. It can infuse into every aspect of your life if you allow it. Mikao Usui Sensei stated that the five Reiki principles are the foundations of the essence of Reiki spiritual practice. However, whether practicing Reiki or not, every person is welcome to incorporate these principles into their lives to attain a soulful and fulfilling life.

As you will see, each principle starts with "just for today." Dr. Usui found that the key to happiness is focusing on the present moment and trying our best every single day. Remember, every day is a fresh start, and you can manage it day by day, wherever you are. Here are each of the five principles, followed by some guidance:

1. **Just for today, I will let go of anger.** It's human to be angry at times; however, notice if you are creating unnecessary suffering for yourself. Remember, letting go of anger at someone does not imply that what they did was okay. Letting go is sometimes about choosing inner peace and acceptance and making room for what awaits you.

2. **Just for today, I will let go of worry.** Trust the unfoldment of your life, even if you don't know what's around the corner. Think of all the times the universe had a way of delivering and circumstances worked in your favor.

3. **Just for today, I will count my blessings.** When you are in a state of gratitude and appreciation, you see the world from a different perspective. What you focus on expands.

4. **Just for today, I will do my work honestly.** Honoring your own values and morals is how you live with purpose. When you do your work honestly and feel good about how you show up in the world, contentment is achieved.

5. **Just for today, I will be kind to every living creature.** Everyone you meet is going through their own battle and trying to navigate life, so extend kindness and compassion for yourself and others. Remember, what goes around, comes around—tenfold.

Three Pillars

Dr. Usui focused on three essential pillars in his Reiki system—Gassho meditation, Reiji-ho, and Chiryo. Let's look at each.

1. **Gassho meditation.** The first pillar of Reiki is Gassho, which translates to "two hands coming together." This is a form of meditation that the Reiki practitioner uses to clear their minds, or ground themselves, before starting the treatment.

   I recommend doing Gassho meditation for about 15 to 30 minutes before each Reiki treatment, as it is a wonderful practice to help you get into a more mindful, centered state before channeling Reiki. Practicing Gassho meditation will also help you clear the mind, open the heart, and purify your vessel before channeling. You can return to Gassho meditation anytime throughout the treatment to feel more grounded and connected.

For this meditation, close your eyes, bring your palms together at your heart center with your thumbs touching your heart, and focus on the space where your middle fingertips meet. Relax, ease into the meditative state, and let the energy flow through you.

2. **Reiji-ho.** The second pillar of Reiki is Reiji-ho, which translates to "indication of the Reiki power methods." During Reiji-ho, you are calling in the Reiki energy and asking Spirit, or Source, for guidance so your hands and Reiki are directed to serve the highest good of the recipient.

    You can say something similar to "I ask that the Reiki be used for the highest good of (*recipient's name*)." You can either ask out loud or in your head, inviting guidance from Spirit.

    After spending several minutes in Gassho meditation, and when you feel that you have connected with Reiki energy through Reiji-ho, bring your hands to your third eye chakra, located between your eyebrows. Give gratitude for this practice, trust that the healing will go where it is needed the most, and allow your hands to be led intuitively.

3. **Chiryo.** The third pillar of Reiki is Chiryo, which translates to "treatment." This pillar refers to the act of laying hands on the body. Reiki is channeled through the practitioner and into the recipient through the hands.

    I recommend beginning the treatment by following your inner guidance and then using the hand position guide in chapter 2 as needed.

The Energy Body

The word *Reiki* translates to "universal life force energy" in Japanese. *Rei* means "universal" or "spiritual," and *ki* means "life force energy." This *ki* is the same thing as *chi* in Chinese medicine, *prana* in Sanskrit, *light* in the Bible, and *dosha* in Ayurvedic medicine. It is the energy that is in each one of us and is responsible for keeping us alive and functioning every day.

You don't have to be spiritual or practice alternative healing to understand that everything in the world is made up of energy, including the human body. The human body is an entwining of subtle energy and a series of complex systems. The energy body is complex and so intelligent that it is constantly rearranging itself to maintain homeostasis—bring the body back to balance.

Our bodies have seven main energy centers along the spine that are known as chakras. *Chakras* translates to "spinning wheel of energy" in Sanskrit, and their purpose is to move and draw in *ki* where it is needed to keep the physical, mental, emotional, and spiritual health of the body in balance.

When *ki* is blocked or constricted around and in the chakras, our well-being is affected in many ways. Reiki can help address an energy block by moving the energy and bringing the body back into alignment. The seven chakras, along with their associations and correspondences, are illustrated in the following figure.

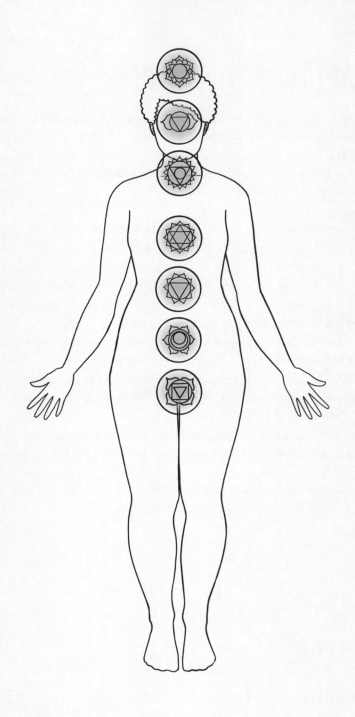

Crown chakra—seventh chakra (violet): Associated with unity consciousness, our connection and relationship to the Divine. Connected to being open spiritually to something greater than ourselves and feeling interconnected with the universe.

Third eye chakra—sixth chakra (indigo): Associated with intuition, awareness, and imagination. Connected to being able to see ourselves clearly and see the world from a more complete perspective.

Throat chakra—fifth chakra (blue): Associated with communication and self-expression. Connected to our ability to speak the truth and communicate authentically.

Heart chakra—fourth chakra (green/pink): Associated with love, acceptance, joy, and compassion. Connected to the quality of our relationships and love of ourselves and others.

Solar plexus chakra—third chakra (yellow): Associated with our self-esteem, self-worth, and boundaries. Connected to our personal power, how we feel about ourselves, and how we interact in the world.

Sacral chakra—second chakra (orange): Associated with our sexuality, pleasure, and creativity. Connected to our ability to express our true emotions and enjoy simple pleasures in our lives.

Root chakra—first chakra (red): Associated with our foundation and basic needs. Connected to our sense of belonging in this world, including security issues and finances.

In-Person Treatment Basics

During a Reiki treatment, use a combination of the hands-on healing technique, Reiki symbols, and your intuition to promote the physical, mental, emotional, and spiritual well-being of the recipient. There is no strict rule when it comes to Reiki, as there are various Reiki techniques and styles that differ according to the practitioner and the lineage they were taught.

When formulating my sessions, I asked myself often, "If I were the one receiving, what would I like to receive in an hour-long Reiki healing treatment? How would I like to feel?" When you are creating your own sessions, think about what you would like to receive yourself, and create exactly that!

Preparing for the Treatment

Here I share what I learned from my teachers and offer a breakdown of steps and best practices for conducting in-person Reiki treatments from beginning to end. If your teacher taught you something that I don't mention, honor what you have been taught. If something I mention is new, try it out to see if it feels good and makes sense to you. Take what resonates, leave what doesn't, and feel free to add your own magic touch to the treatment to make it yours. My sequence for in-person treatment begins with the following basic steps.

1. SPACE

Create a space that invites warmth and serenity. Spend some time making sure the space you are practicing in is physically clean and decluttered. Remember, the goal is to help the recipient feel good and grounded in this space. Here are a few guidelines:

- Set up a comfortable space for the recipient to lie on such as a massage table; you can also use a bed, sofa, or floor with cushions. Feel free to lay out blanket, pillow, and an eye mask.

- Dim the lights and burn some naturally scented candles to set the mood and generate a pleasant smell.

- Play calming, healing music in the background—that is, your favorite meditative music that makes you feel at ease. I recommend making your own playlist for your Reiki treatments because it's a lot of fun. I use Spotify, but you can also look up "Reiki music" on YouTube and find plenty of free resources.

2. CLEANSE + PROTECT

Burn your favorite nonendangered, dried plant or natural incense to purify your space and transmute negative or stagnant energy. Cultures from all over the world have used sacred plants for thousands of years to cleanse people and spaces of negativity and promote healing. When you are choosing a plant for cleansing, purchase only from sellers who source their products sustainably and ethically. Growing your own plant is a wonderful idea too. When you are burning these plants or incense, keep at least one window open, as it's important that the energy you are removing has a pathway to escape.

If you don't want to participate in the smoke-cleansing ritual, that's okay too. If you received second-degree Reiki training, you could

beam the Power Symbol (Cho Ku Rei; see page 83) to the four corners of the room to cleanse and protect your space. To do so, invoke
the symbol by drawing it in the air and direct your hands to "send it"
toward each of the four corners. If you received your third-degree
Reiki training, you could beam the Master Symbol (Dai Ko Myo; see
page 86) to the four corners of the room instead.

Travel tip: You can use the beaming symbol technique to cleanse,
protect, and bless any space or room. I personally like to do this
when staying at hotels or vacation rentals. Imagine how many
people stayed in that same space! This is a great technique for
empaths who travel often and feel other people's energies easily.

3. GASSHO MEDITATION

Practice Gassho meditation for at least 15 minutes before you start the
treatment. I like to do this before the recipient walks into the room so
that I can connect to the energy of Reiki before meeting the person.
You can also do this in the beginning of a treatment while you are
with the recipient.

Note: Practices like meditation and breathwork are not essential
for Reiki to succeed, but I've found that these practices create a
nice flow leading up to Reiki. I describe receiving Reiki as similar to
getting ready for sleep. For example, when you are getting ready
for bed, you brush your teeth, change into comfortable pajamas,
turn off the lights, etc. Those things are not necessarily essential for
you to fall asleep, but they sure do help you fall asleep faster. Your
job as a Reiki practitioner is to help the recipient obtain a more
open and receptive state by creating an environment that will help
them break free from their logical mind and stay present in their
bodies and hearts so that Reiki can be received and felt.

Connecting with the Recipient

Before every treatment, I get to know the recipient and discuss their specific concerns, goals, or intentions, if any. This is a good time to explain Reiki if it's their first time as a recipient and share what to expect during your Reiki treatment. Build rapport with the recipient so they feel comfortable with you and safe in your company.

If they don't know what they are aiming to receive from treatment, that's okay too. You may want to offer a few prompts to get a sense of how they feel and what they are working to heal, such as:

- *What is one thing that hasn't been working?*

- *What is one thing that has been working?*

- *What do you need more of in this moment?*

- *What do you feel in this moment?*

- *What is one thing you want to release going forward?*

- *What is one thing you want to make room for going forward?*

Sometimes we don't know what we need and the best way to receive Reiki is to start with an open mind and consider what surfaces during the treatment.

Starting and Ending Treatments

You don't have to adhere to the exact steps listed here for Reiki to start flowing, and you might have learned some variations. Some practitioners simply say, "Please allow Reiki to flow wherever it is needed for the highest and greatest good," and then start channeling right away. I participate in the following steps because it helps me connect to the Reiki energy more powerfully and keeps me mindful while practicing.

1. Draw the Power Symbol (Cho Ku Rei; see page 83) on your palms and then bring your hands to your heart center and then to your third eye chakra.

2. Reiji-ho: Ask Spirit and your Reiki guides to help lead you to the areas that need most healing. I like to call on the Reiki teachers who have come before us for their blessing and protection. I say something such as "Dr. Usui, Dr. Hayashi Sensei, and Mrs. Takata, calling in the Reiki energies for the highest good and individual healing for *(recipient's name).*"

3. Draw a big Power Symbol above the recipient's body to start.

4. Beam all three symbols into their crown chakra while chanting the recipient's name.

5. Treat the body using your intuition and the hand position guide (see chapter 2) along with the Reiki symbols for which you received attunements/placements during training.

6. When you are ready to end the treatment, invoke a big Power Symbol above the recipient's body to seal in the treatment.

7. Give gratitude for the practice. I like to seal the treatment by saying, "Dr. Usui, Dr. Hayashi, and Mrs. Takata, calling in the Reiki energy for the highest good and individual healing for *(recipient's name)*. Thank you." I say it out loud to let the recipient know that the treatment is almost at its end.

8. Ask your guides if there is anything they want you to share with the recipient and, if so, share it.

9. Cleanse the recipient's energetic field by placing your hands a few inches above their head and stroking them down all the way to the bottom of their feet, as if you are sweeping. Repeat 2 more times.

10. Let the recipient know the treatment is over and that you will leave the room to give them some privacy and will return in about five minutes.

11. In the other room, do Kenyoku (see the steps and illustrations to follow) to cleanse your energetic field and then wash your hands.

12. Return to the room and ask the recipient to share their experience with you.

Kenyoku

Kenyoku is a practice you can incorporate both before and after your treatment to cleanse your energetic field, removing any unwanted energy that is not yours. You can consider Kenyoku a form of spiritual hygiene. I cleanse my aura both before I start and after I finish a treatment. Here's how:

1. Place your right hand on top of your left shoulder.

2. Brush your hand down diagonally all the way to the bottom of your right hip. Flick your wrist as if you are shaking something off your hand.

3. Place your left hand on top of your right shoulder.

4. Brush your hand down diagonally all the way to the bottom of your left hip. Flick your wrist as if you are shaking something off your hand. Repeat once more on each side.

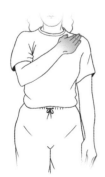 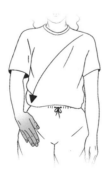 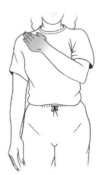 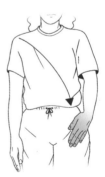

5. Place your right hand on top of your left shoulder.

6. Brush your right hand all the way down your left arm to your fingertips. Flick your wrist.

7. Place your left hand on top of your right shoulder.

8. Brush your left hand all the way down your right arm to your fingertip. Flick your wrist. Repeat once more on each side.

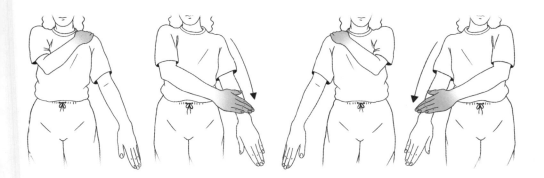

Distant Reiki

Although Reiki is often carried out with an in-person, hands-on treatment, it can also be practiced over distance and time. After receiving your second-degree Reiki attunement, you can use the Distant Symbol (Hon Sha Ze Sho Nen; see page 85) to send Reiki to people you are not physically with. And because energy is not limited by distance and time, it can be sent to heal past and future events.

I was skeptical of distant healing at first and wondered how Reiki could possibly work if the practitioner is not physically with the recipient. It's normal and smart to question these kinds of ideas, and I highly recommend trying both giving and receiving distant Reiki to find out for yourself.

Many Reiki practitioners believe distant Reiki works because we all originate from Source, where all energy is one and energy transcends space and time. Because of this, we are all interconnected and can communicate and link up energetically with one another without using verbal communication and across great distances.

For example, have you ever thought of someone randomly and they call you the next minute, or you dream about someone and run into them the next day? Or you are sending distant Reiki to a recipient with a knee injury and suddenly feel tension in your knees too? I believe we can feel a person's energy even if they're not physically present, because energy is not bound by time or space. I know this might be hard to wrap your head around at first, but I strongly encourage you to get out of your logical mind and start practicing. It's one of those concepts you can't really explain but can feel.

Benefits of Distant Reiki

Doing Reiki over distances has wonderful benefits, including:

- The recipient can receive healing in the comfort of their home. This is great for people who have busy schedules or cannot travel.

- When people who are skeptical of energy healing feel the effects of distant healing from miles away, they become more trusting and open to alternative healing modalities such as Reiki.

- Holding distant Reiki sessions opens you up to clientele from all over the world because you are not limited to people in your town, city, or state. There are 7.9 billion people in the world today—remember this if you ever think there are too many Reiki practitioners or the field is too competitive. In fact, most of my income is from distant Reiki sessions and my virtual Reiki certification courses.

- When you hold distant Reiki treatments for people you never met in person, you learn to appreciate more accurate and unbiased, intuitive messages during Gassho meditation and Chiryo (see "Developing Intuition with Distant Reiki" on page 35).

- This is a wonderful way to time travel to the past or future to either heal inner child and past traumas or empower future goals and dreams.

Distant Reiki Techniques

There are various techniques you can use when practicing distant Reiki. I personally use a combination of Enkaku Chiryo, a stuffed animal, and crystals to help me visualize and connect with the person to which I am sending healing. No technique is more effective than the other, so use what feels natural to you. Let's look at each.

ENKAKU CHIRYO

Enkaku translates to "sending," and *Chiryo* translates to "treatment." For this technique, get a picture of the recipient or write their name on a piece of paper. Alternatively, perform the treatment over live video; have the recipient lie down far enough from the camera so that their whole body, from head to toe, fits in the screen. Follow these steps:

1. Draw the Power Symbol (Cho Ku Rei; see page 83) on both of your palms.

2. Place the picture or piece of paper between your hands and enter Gassho meditation (see page 13) with your thumbs touching your heart. You can place the picture or paper in front of you and beam your hands from a distance.

3. Perform Reiji-ho (see page 14).

4. Invoke the Distant Symbol (Hon Sha Ze Sho Nen; see page 85) either by drawing it in the air, visualizing it in your head, or saying "Hon Sha Ze Sho Nen" three times.

5. Assume a meditative state and allow Reiki to flow toward the person you are healing. Visualize Reiki entering the recipient from the crown chakra and filling up their entire body—from head to toe. Use any other symbols during the treatment that you feel inclined to use.

SURROGATE METHOD

In this technique, use a stuffed animal as a surrogate to represent the person to whom you will be sending Reiki. For hand position purposes, be sure the stuffed animal has a head, two legs, and two arms to mirror the human anatomy. For example, a teddy bear is a better fit than a stuffed dolphin. You can proceed with the treatment as if the teddy bear were the recipient. Follow these steps:

1. Draw the Power Symbol (Cho Ku Rei; see page 83) on both of your palms and come into Gassho meditation.

2. Perform Reiji-ho (see page 14).

3. Say, "As I give a Reiki treatment to this stuffed animal, I am giving a session to *(recipient's name)*."

4. Invoke the Distant Symbol (Hon Sha Ze Sho Nen; see page 85).

5. Using a combination of your intuition and the hand positions, give the stuffed animal a complete treatment, as if the toy were actually the recipient.

CRYSTALS

Crystals are known to carry special healing elements and properties and work as conduits for natural healing energy. They can also work as a conduit and bridge between the practitioner and recipient during distant healing treatments. Follow these steps:

1. Print an outline of the human figure (see the following image).

2. Designate one crystal for each of the seven chakras (see page 17) and lay them out along the figure's spine. You can pair up the crystal and the chakra based on color (for example, a red crystal for the root chakra), but rely on your intuition to make the choice.

3. Draw the Power Symbol (Cho Ku Rei; see page 83) on both of your palms and come into Gassho meditation.

4. Perform Reiji-ho (see page 14).

5. Invoke the Distant Symbol (Hon Sha Ze Sho Nen; see page 85).

6. Start channeling distant Reiki and beam Reiki to each crystal and its corresponding chakra one at a time—either by holding the crystal between your hands or holding your hands a few inches above the crystal.

Optional: If you work with pendulums, you can hover the pendulum over each crystal to determine which chakra is open or blocked. Spend additional time beaming Reiki on the crystal representing the blocked chakra.

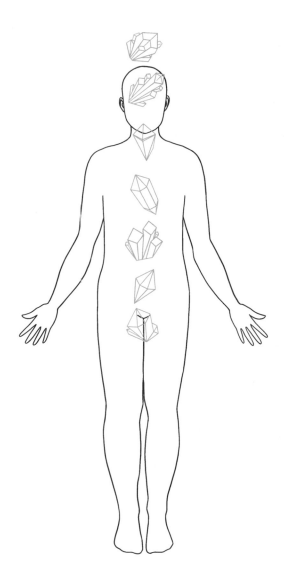

DISTANT REIKI TREATMENT BASICS

When sending distant Reiki to someone, you should ask them for their permission. For distant treatments, I highly recommend setting up a time that works for both you and them, a time when they can find a quiet, comfortable place to sink into the experience.

Sessions can be performed over the phone or by video chat. For professional sessions, I like to have one-to-one interaction with the recipient and touch base before and after the treatment. I send distant Reiki off-line, but you can stay on the phone or keep your video on for the whole session. If you choose to send Reiki off-line, ask the recipient to put their phone on airplane mode and set a timer for the length of your session. Then, when the timer sounds, ask them to call you back to reconnect. Be sure to set your timer as well.

From holding hundreds of distant Reiki treatments over the years, I have formulated a sequence that flows very beautifully. This sequence is similar to my sequence for in-person treatment (see page 18), with a few minor differences. Feel free to incorporate any other practices from your healing toolbox to the sequence and modify as needed. This is just what has worked for me! Remember, healing is an art. Create a treatment sequence that feels natural and unique to you.

PREPARING FOR THE TREATMENT

As soon as a client confirms a booking, I send out an email with all the details they will need. Instead of preparing the room, I ask them to set up a sacred space prior to the treatment because I cannot be with them physically. My email generally looks something like this:

Hi *(insert client's name)*,

I will be calling you on *(insert date and time)* for our distant Reiki session.

To save time and to get the most out of our time together, I highly recommend you do the following prior to the session:

- Set up a comfortable spot either on your bed or the floor where you can relax and be undisturbed for a whole hour. Grab your favorite blanket, pillow, and eye mask to make it a relaxing experience.
- Have a laptop nearby and pull up this music link to play in the background at the start of our session: *(insert URL to healing music you like on YouTube)*. It would be best if you play it from your laptop so the sound doesn't interfere with our phone call.
- Wear your most comfortable clothes, drink a lot of water, and try your best to eat light that day.

Please reply to this email with:

- A few sentences explaining what you are looking to gain from our session together. It can be anything physical, emotional, mental, or spiritual.
- The best number to reach you on the day of our session.

Looking forward to our session together!
All the best,
Hae

On the day of the treatment, spend at least 15 minutes in Gassho meditation before calling the recipient. Bring out the healing tools— that is, crystals and body outline, photo or paper and pen, or stuffed animal—depending on the technique you choose.

CONNECTING WITH THE RECIPIENT

Call the recipient and give them a quick rundown of how your sessions will proceed. This is also a good time to review their response to your email and ask them to share their goals and intentions for the session. Instruct them to click on the music link you emailed them and play it in the background.

Lead a guided meditation of your choosing to help them become grounded and open. You don't know what the person was doing prior to the session, so try to incorporate practices that will help them feel relaxed before they go into the treatment. I usually do either an inner child past or future meditation, depending on what the client is confronting.

I do a few rounds of the 4-7-8 breathwork technique with the recipient for 60 seconds. This technique works as a natural tranquilizer for the nervous system. It should put the recipient in a more relaxed state. Instruct them as follows:

1. Inhale through your nose to a count of four.

2. Hold your breath for a count of seven.

3. Exhale through your mouth for a count of eight.

4. Repeat.

After the breathwork exercise, ask the recipient to breathe deeply in through their nose and out through their mouth throughout the rest of the treatment.

STARTING AND ENDING TREATMENT

1. Send Reiki to the recipient using any of the distant Reiki techniques (see page 32) for the length of the session.

2. When the session is over, ask the recipient how they feel and if they would like to share anything with you about their Reiki journey. Feel free to share any insights you encountered during the treatment and Gassho meditation.

3. Following the call, perform Kenyoku (see page 24) to cleanse your energetic field.

4. Email the recipient to say thank you and summarize the main takeaways from the session. This follow-up email is a great opportunity to build rapport and inform them of your offerings and events or request testimonials.

Developing Intuition with Distant Reiki

Regardless of your spiritual beliefs, you have likely experienced a time in your life when your intuition was accurate even though logical, conscious reasoning couldn't support your gut feeling. I believe that every single one of us is intuitive, but developing our intuition is like working a muscle. We are all born with muscles, but it's up to each individual to develop and strengthen them; the same goes for intuition.

A famous author and speaker in the fields of self-development and spiritual growth Wayne Dyer once said, "If prayers is you talking to God, then intuition is God talking to you." I believe that our intuition is always communicating with us, but we must quiet our minds, declutter outside noise, and get into a receptive state to be able to receive the message. When we quiet our mind, intuition can flow in like a river.

A wonderful aspect about holding distant Reiki sessions is that it helps you strengthen your intuitive muscle over time. When you are holding treatments for people you know little about, the information you "receive" turns out to be more unbiased and accurate. For example, when you see someone in person, your mind can unconsciously start gathering information based on what they look like, what they're wearing, the energy they carry coming into the room, etc. When this happens, your logical mind might interfere with your intuition. Therefore, to strengthen your intuition, I highly recommend spending as much time as you can in Gassho meditation before calling the recipient. Notice if you perceive any information about them during your meditation. This may arise as visuals, repeated thoughts, sounds, feelings, or simply a knowing.

When I first started holding distant Reiki sessions, I realized that I would sense a lot of imagery and random words during my Gassho meditation. I had many instances where I felt the need to share with my client, and my clients often reported back to me that my message was exactly what they needed to hear. For example, I kept hearing the word "sprouts" during my Gassho meditation for a client, and my mind immediately thought of the organic grocery store chain by the same name. I also saw a visual of a big farm. When my client spoke on the phone, she mentioned that she was an accountant, so I didn't know how this information was relevant. I decided to share it anyway.

She thanked me and said she'd been thinking about quitting her accounting job to travel and partake in Worldwide Opportunities on Organic Farms (WWOOF, a community exchange program that connects visitors with organic farmers for educational immersion around the world). She was scared to leave what was familiar to her and had been looking for a big sign—and this was it. She emailed me a few months later to thank me for relaying that confirmation to her, because it nudged her to pursue her dream.

If you do not receive any information about the person during meditation and treatment, this doesn't mean you are doing something wrong. Our job as Reiki healers is not to diagnose or predict anyone's future or tell them what to do, by any means. Yet, sometimes we are nudged to share some information with the person, and it's okay to share and co-create the significance of the message, as long as you believe that the message is for their highest good and your ego is not involved.

Self-Treatments, Reiki for Animals, and More

There are so many wonderful ways to incorporate Reiki into your daily life. Let's look at how to use Reiki for yourself, animals, and elements in nature, and how one can imbue objects with Reiki.

Self-Treatments

After receiving first-degree Reiki training, you can start giving yourself Reiki, which is a wonderful way to become familiar with this practice. I highly recommend practicing Reiki on yourself as an act of self-love before you practice on others; this way, you can first replenish your own energy source, experience Reiki firsthand, and feel more connected to Source.

Practicing Reiki on yourself has many benefits. Reiki can be used as a self-soothing technique whenever you are anxious or stressed, as it promotes feelings of peace, gratitude, and love. It can be used to heal physical, emotional, or mental pain or to strengthen your immune system when your body is feeling out of balance. It is also known to help with your personal and spiritual growth, as this practice often reveals your authentic self (who you are at your core) and can divulge patterns on which you need to manage and heal. It can also be used to eliminate blocks and negativity within your energy system, help with your personal problems, and cultivate awareness to remove whatever is obstructing your goals.

The length of the self-treatment depends on you and your schedule. You can give yourself a complete treatment, doing the hand positions from head to toe (see chapter 2). If you are short on time, though, you can focus on specific areas and rely on your intuition to determine where to place your hands. Remember, there is no wrong way to give yourself love and appreciation.

You can do a Reiki self-treatment whenever and wherever you feel inclined, but I personally love practicing right after I wake up, to set a positive mood for the rest of the day, or right before I go to bed, to prepare for a restful sleep. The most important element is that you feel grounded and relaxed and choose a time and place that feels comfortable for you.

You can use the self-treatment hand positions as a guide along with your intuition when treating yourself. I usually spend about three to five minutes per hand position, but you can do it for however long you feel is needed. If you don't know where to start, placing one hand over your heart and the other on your stomach is a great beginning. Connecting to the rhythm of your breath in this way is very grounding.

Experiment and try all the hand positions so you know what they feel like; this can tell you how much pressure and distance to use when you are treating others. It also allows room to be creative with the hand positions and even create positions that are not included in chapter 2, as you will discover which hand positions feel effective and natural to you.

For self-treatments, I do not engage in any complicated steps before I start channeling. I try my best to achieve a receptive state so I can quiet the mental chatter and come into my heart for Reiki to flow through me. I play relaxing music in the background, set an intention, say something such as "allow Reiki to flow wherever is needed for the highest and greatest good," and then intuitively place my hands to wherever I am drawn.

Sending Reiki to Animals

If you have pets, you might have noticed that they love being in your presence during your Reiki attunements and treatments. Animals are energy-receptive beings and are magnetized to this healing, relaxing energy. All animals can benefit from Reiki just as much as humans do. Here's how Reiki can help animals:

- Strengthens connection and communication between pet and owner

- Reduces anxiety

- Comforts animals who have undergone trauma or abuse

- Speeds up recovery from injuries and surgery

- Assists in end-of-life support

- Assists in emotional healing

When treating animals, I recommend beaming Reiki across the room first and then slowly approaching the animal so you can get a sense of how they are responding. If the animal desires a direct inter-action, they will come closer to you. If not, you can beam Reiki from afar or even use one of the distant Reiki techniques (see page 32).

If the animal is your pet or knows you well, they might feel comfortable to lie down and position themselves to tell you where exactly Reiki is needed and where to place your hands.

As for hand positions, I mostly rely on my intuition and place my hands where I think the animal would feel the most comfortable. You may choose to refer to the hand position guide in chapter 2 and adapt and modify as you proceed. Of course, if there is a specific injury, place your hands either very lightly over or beam a few inches above the wounded area. Use your best judgment.

If you want to work with a specific type of animal, spend some time learning the anatomy of that animal. If you want to work mainly with animals, you can take a course on animal Reiki. I recommend visiting the International Center for Reiki Training website (Reiki.org) for more information.

Sending Reiki to Nature

Have you ever sat silently and watched the leaves of a tree swaying in the wind, and it feels as if they are whispering to you? You see firsthand that the trees are breathing, living beings just like you are and that the divinity in them is also in you. Divinity is found in all things on this earthly world, so I highly recommend sharing Reiki with anything in nature—including plants, trees, clouds, the sky, bodies of water, and mountains—and notice how peaceful and connected you feel. You will not only understand but also feel that you are one with Mother Nature.

Many people experiment sharing Reiki with their houseplants. Plants have been shown to sense and respond to certain vibrations. People even believe that plants grow faster when you talk to them. To me, it totally makes sense, as I believe that any living thing will respond positively to love, care, and attention. Considering that plants respond to vibrations, you can be sure that they will love some Reiki from you!

Imbuing Reiki into Objects

You can turn any ordinary object into a sacred object by imbuing Reiki into it. You can also send Reiki to anything material—a house, car, laptop, painting, book, pencil, etc., and bless it with Reiki. You can do this by either holding the object in your hands or directing your hands a few inches away from the object to fill the item with Reiki. I like to meditate with the object in my hand, set a specific intention, and ask the object to be filled with positive, healing energies.

Imbuing crystals with Reiki is common because most crystals have extraordinary abilities to store, transmit, and transform *energy and intention*. Crystals have the unique ability to hold consciousness and will continue to send Reiki even after you are done beaming Reiki into it.

You can imbue Reiki into crystals and gift them to people you want to send continuous healing to but can't be with physically. For example, when my grandmother had stage 4 cancer during the COVID-19 pandemic, I could only see her for a few minutes at a time. Because I couldn't be by her side, I spent days meditating and imbuing Reiki into one crystal and gave it to her to hold onto while she slept. Consider this the next time you want to send healing to someone you can't be with in person. Pick a sacred object that means a lot to you. Carry it around with you for a couple of days and send Reiki to it. Then, gift it to your loved one.

CHAPTER TWO

Hand Positions

This chapter describes and illustrates hand positions for treating others as well as yourself. These hand positions are guidelines for you to follow as needed. You don't have to use every hand position for a session to be considered a complete treatment. You might feel inclined to skip a few hand positions, spend more time on specific areas of the body, or change the order of the positions along the way.

Hand Positions for Treating Others

I recommend using these positions as a starting point and allowing your intuition to lead your hands. As you gain more experience, your intuition might even lead you to treat areas that are not mentioned here. For example, position 2 for eyes and position 3 for chest/heart are positions I intuitively came up with over the years. Remember, healing is an art, and there is no one-size-fits-all approach when it comes to Reiki.

Most Reiki practitioners start the treatment at the top of the head and make their way down to the feet. I personally save the hand positions for the feet until the end of the session to keep my hands clean for the rest of the body.

Here are a few things to note before you start the treatment:

- Set aside at least five minutes to explore why the recipient sought out Reiki and what they hope to achieve through treatment. For example, if they are coming in for an elbow injury, you will naturally spend more time around the elbows.

- Ask the recipient permission to directly lay your hands on their body. Explain that Reiki works just as effectively when the hands are a few inches away from the body, but hands-on treatments often help people feel more relaxed because they feel held and comforted.

- Always beam Reiki three to four inches away from the body when working on the throat/neck, breasts, and pelvic area.

- Try to keep your hands as steady as possible if you choose to directly lay your hands on the body. When switching hand positions, do it gently and carefully. You can either sit on a chair, rest your knees on a cushion, or stand firmly to prevent your hands from shaking. If you naturally have shaky hands, I recommend beaming Reiki a few inches away from the body instead, as trembling hands can make the recipient feel uneasy.

- I recommend spending at least three minutes on each hand position; although, the length may vary depending on each recipient and how you feel throughout the treatment.

- Halfway through the session, you can have the recipient turn over onto their stomach and treat the backside of the body, but it's not always necessary. Of course, if a recipient came in for a back problem specifically, you would have the recipient lie on their stomach and you would lay your hands around the back area. I personally don't treat most people on their stomach because I found that the person is usually in such a deep relaxed state that asking them to turn over halfway through the treatment usually wakes them up and disrupts their harmony. But, as always, follow your intuition. Remember, Reiki flows to places beyond where your hands are and travels to the area that needs the most healing.

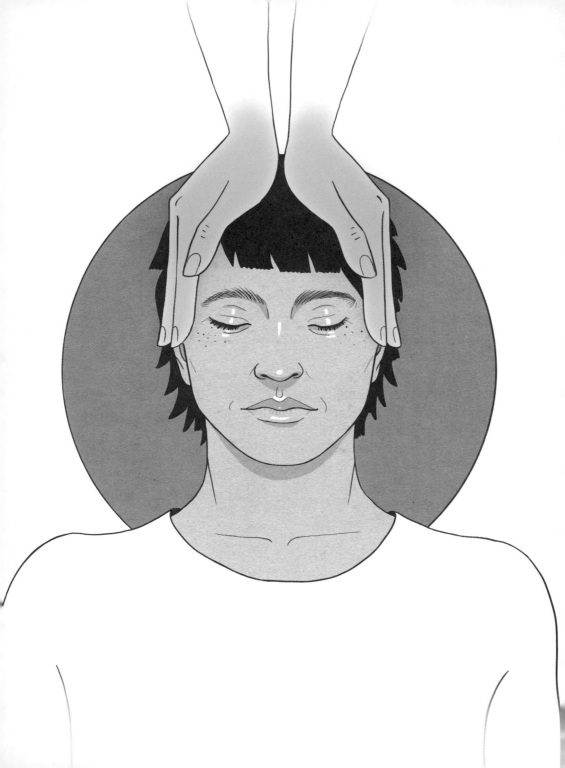

Head

1. Stand or sit above the recipient's head. Cup your hands, touch your wrists together, and gently place the base of your hands at the top of the head with your fingers extending toward each temple.

2. Ask the recipient to gently lift their head, and then place your hands beneath the head, palms facing up with your fingertips touching the base of the skull. Hold the head as if you are cradling a baby.

    These head positions often bring out the feelings of warmth and tenderness as the recipient feels held and supported. When you are ready to go to the next position, slowly and gently remove your hands while supporting the head.

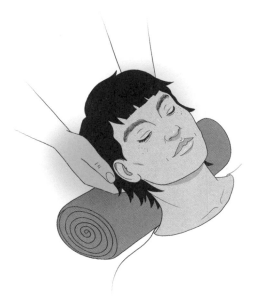

Ears

Place your cupped hands over each side of the ears, with your finger-tips touching, pointing toward the shoulders.

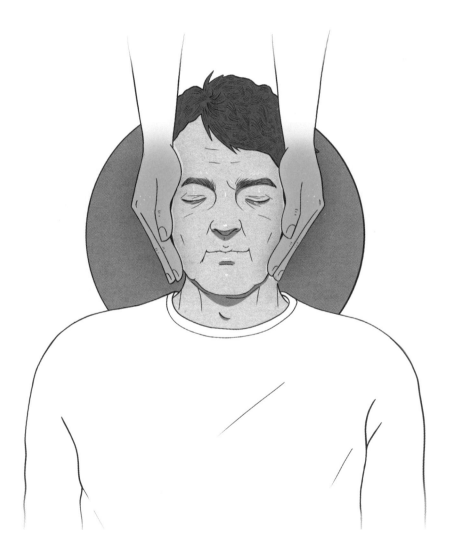

Eyes

At the beginning of the session, I usually place an eye mask on the recipient's eyes to promote relaxation. If you use an eye mask, place it aside for these hand positions.

1. Hover your cupped hands a few inches above the eyes, so that the palms of your hands are not touching the face. You can gently rest the base of your hands on the top of the forehead and keep your fingers away from the face. Make sure not to hover over the recipient's nostrils to avoid constricting their breathing.

2. You may be inclined to carefully place your index, middle, and ring fingers on top of each eyelid with very little to no pressure. Your fingers should be barely touching the eyelids. If you don't have steady hands, I recommend hovering your fingers about three to four inches away.

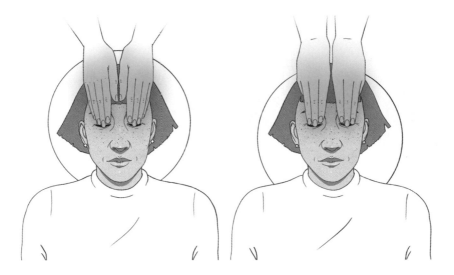

Neck/Throat

Remember, do not directly touch the neck/throat area because this is a very sensitive area for many people. Even if the recipient gave you permission to perform the hands-on positions, I recommend hovering about three to four inches away when treating this area.

1. Hover your hands around each side of the neck, with your fingertips pointing toward the shoulders.

2. From behind the recipient's head, make a V shape with your index fingers pointing toward each other. Hover your hands over the collarbone. Be careful not to touch the throat.

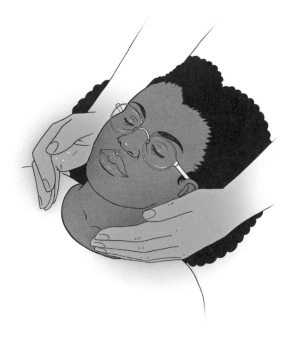

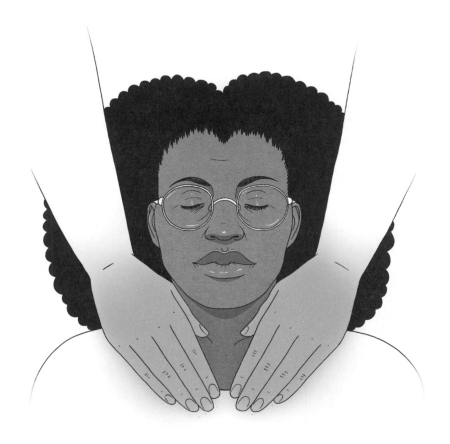

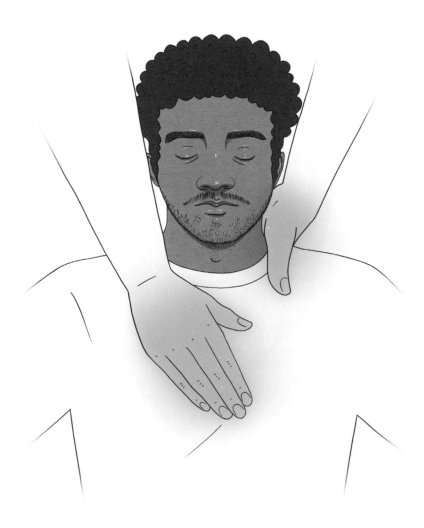

Chest/Heart

When working with the chest/heart area, use your best judgment and make sure you do not directly touch the breasts. In this case, you can beam Reiki three to four inches above the heart. You can choose one or combine any of the following positions:

1. Place your left hand under the neck and gently hover your right hand a few inches above the heart.

2. Stand beside the recipient. Place one hand diagonally in front of the other and hover them a few inches above the heart.

3. Have the recipient place one hand over their heart and the other one on their stomach. Place your hands directly on top of the recipient's hands.

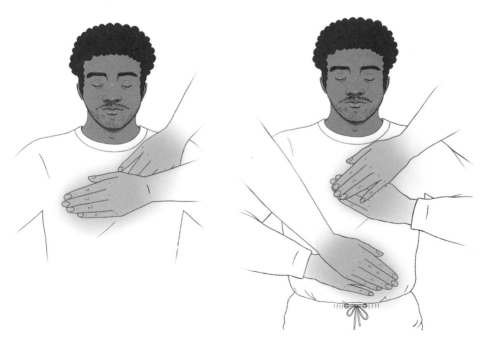

Upper Abdomen

Put one hand diagonally in front of the other and place them on the upper abdomen along the ribs.

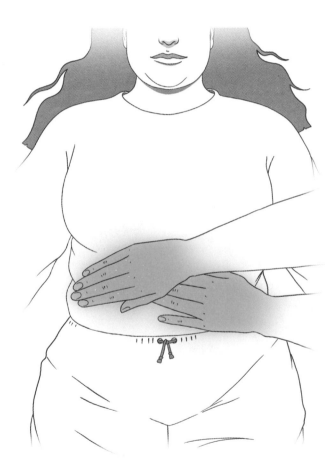

Middle Abdomen

Place one hand on top of the belly button and the other hand below the belly button.

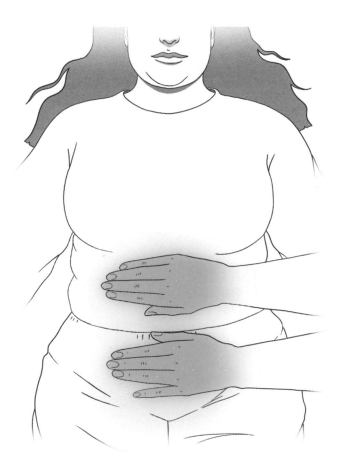

Lower Abdomen

Put one hand diagonally in front of the other and place them across the waistline.

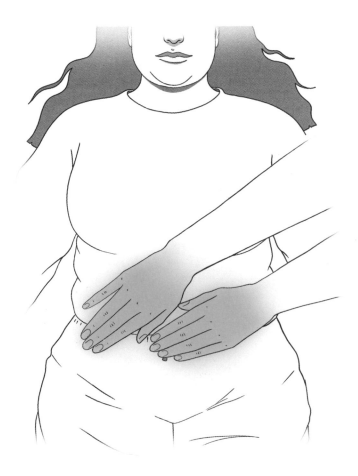

Pelvic Area

Put one hand diagonally in front of the other and hover your hands across the pelvic area just above the pubic bone, a few inches away from the body.

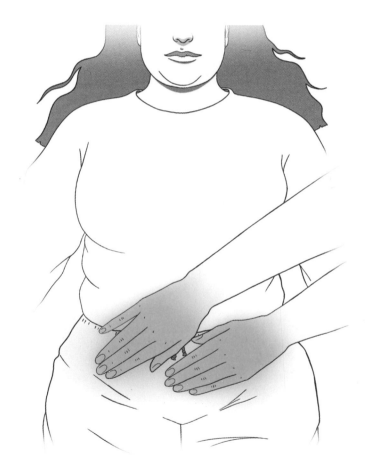

Knees

Stand beside the recipient and place one hand on top of each kneecap.

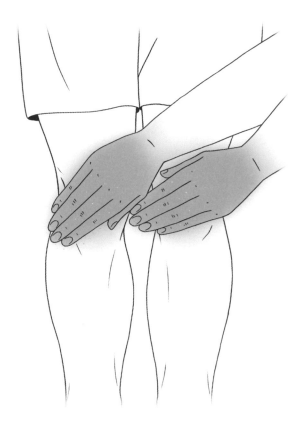

Ankles

1. Stand below the feet. Gently wrap your hands around each ankle.

2. Stand beside the recipient. Wrap one hand around one side of the ankle and the other hand around the other side of the ankle.

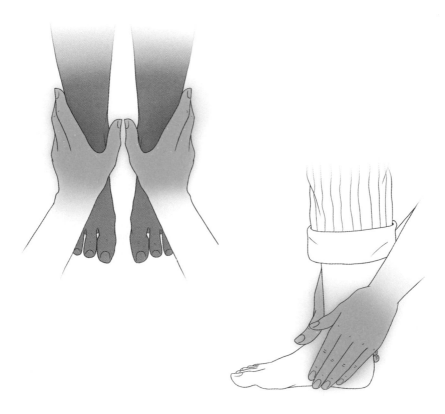

Feet

I recommend asking the recipient to take their socks and shoes off and directly touching the skin. Skin-to-skin contact around the feet feels very grounding, balancing, and anchoring. Make sure to wash your hands after touching the feet.

1. Hold one foot with both hands, one hand on top of the foot and the other one at the sole of the foot. You might be directed to gently massage the soles of the feet. Repeat on the other foot.

2. Place one hand on each sole of the feet. Place your thumbs in the center of the middle area and wrap the rest of the fingers around the feet.

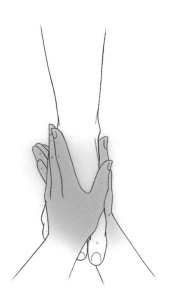
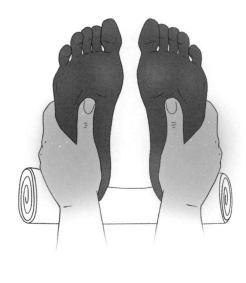

Shoulders (on Stomach)

Stand beside the recipient and place one hand on top of each shoulder.

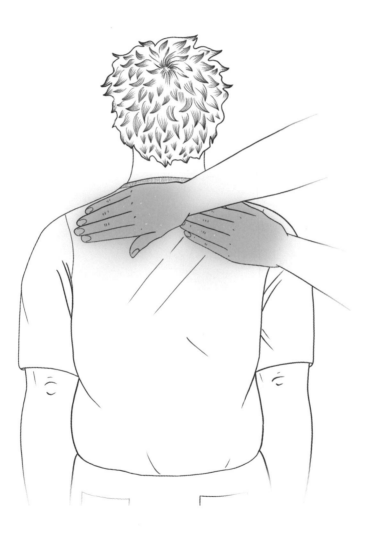

Middle Back (on Stomach)

Stand beside the recipient and place both of your hands across the middle back area, touching the bottom of the shoulder blades.

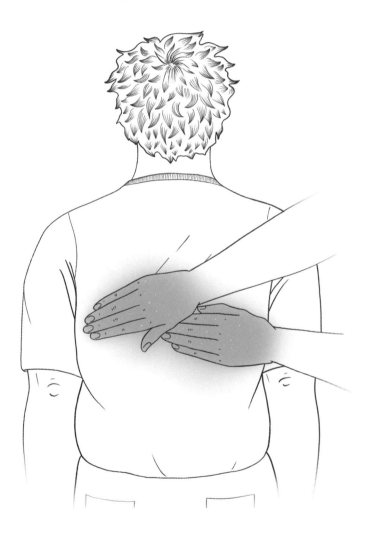

Lower Back (on Stomach)

Stand beside the recipient and place both of your hands across the waist area.

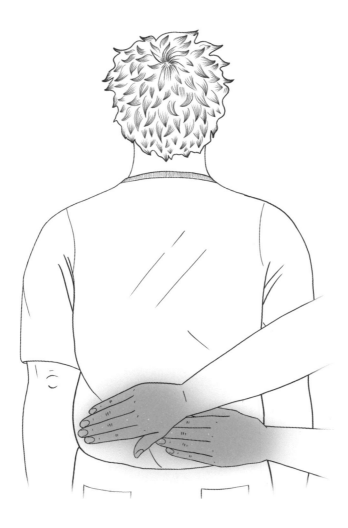

Hand Positions for Self-Treatments

Again, I recommend using these positions as a starting point and allowing your intuition to lead your hands. As you gain more experience, your intuition might even indicate to treat areas that are not mentioned here. When doing the positions for the upper half of your body, you can either lie down on a comfortable bed or couch or sit up. For the bottom half, sit up.

Head

1. Place your hands on top of your head with your middle fingers pointing toward each other.

2. Place your hands on the back of your head with your fingers pointing up.

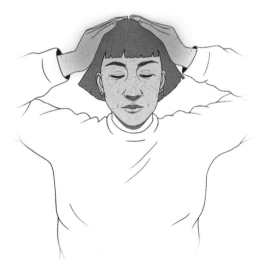
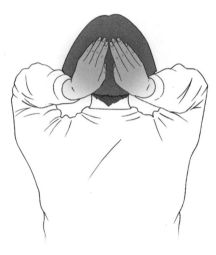

Ears

Cup your hands and place one over each ear.

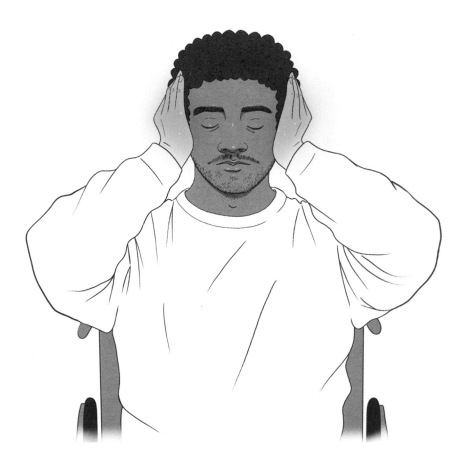

Eyes

1. Cup your hands and place the palms over your eyes with your fingers extending toward the forehead.

2. Place your index, middle, and ring finger on top of each eyelid.

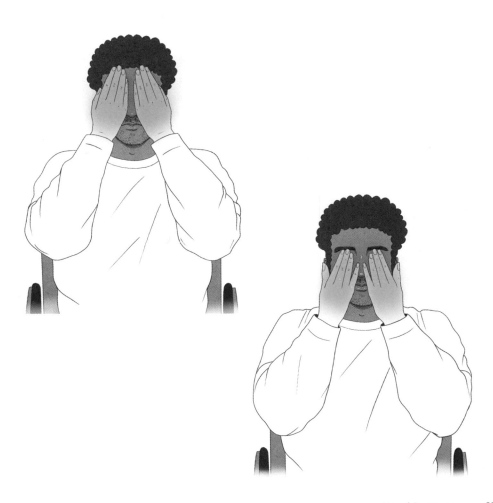

Throat

1. Cup your hands and place them on each side of your neck.

2. Place your left hand over your throat and your right hand over your heart.

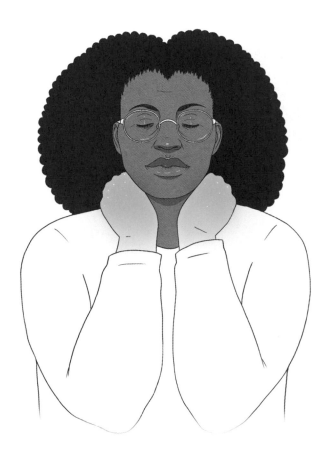

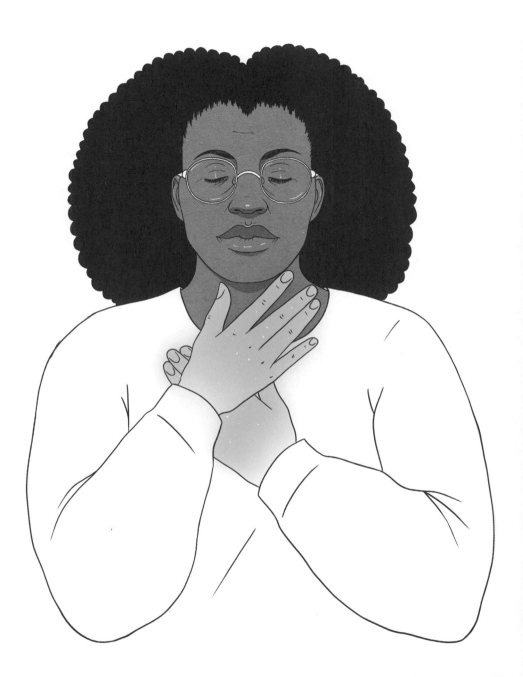

Shoulders

Place your hands over your shoulders with your fingers pointing to your back.

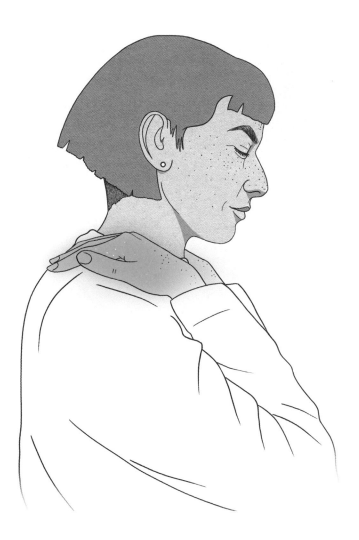

Chest/Heart

1. Place your hands over your heart with your middle fingers pointing toward each other.

2. Place your left hand over your heart and your right hand on your stomach.

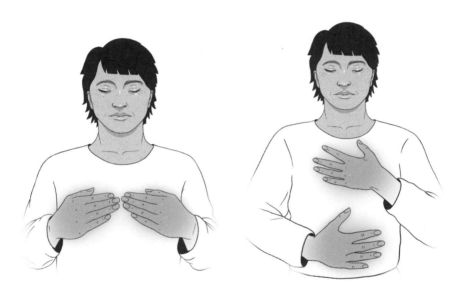

Upper Abdomen

Place your hands over your upper stomach just below your chest with your middle fingers pointing toward each other.

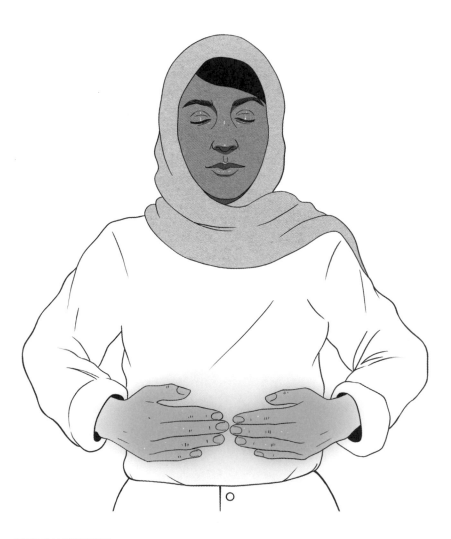

Middle Abdomen

Place your hands on top of your stomach with your middle fingers pointing toward each other on top of your belly button.

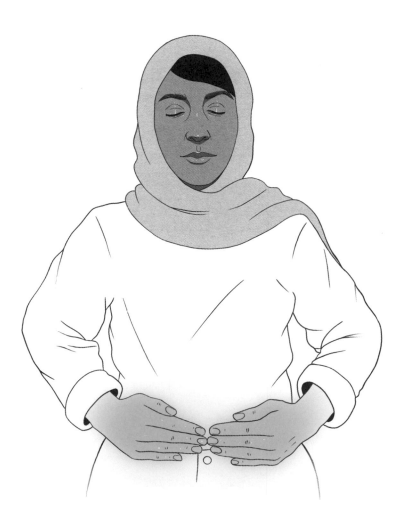

Lower Abdomen

Make a V shape with your hands and place the base of your hands on top of your hip bones with your fingers extending along your pubic bone.

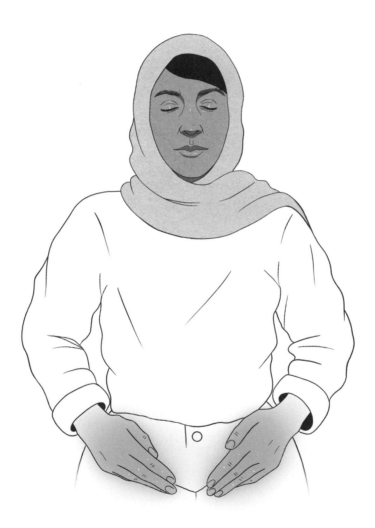

Middle Back

Place your hands on your middle back with your middle fingers pointing toward each other.

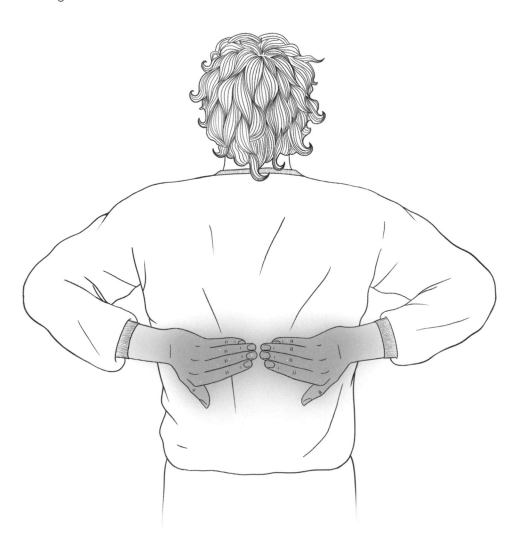

Lower Back

Place your hands on your lower back, across your waistline, with your middle fingers pointing toward each other.

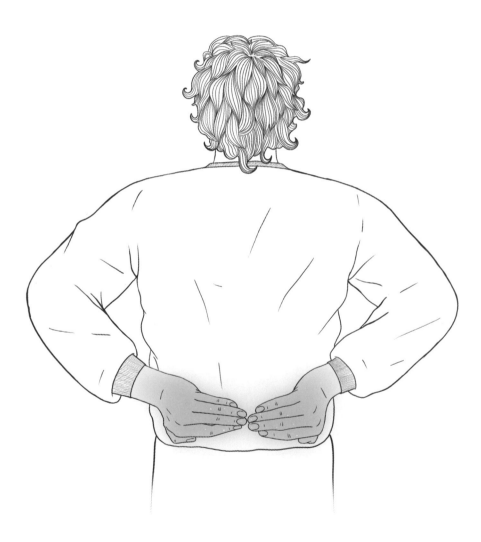

Knees

Place your hands directly over your kneecaps.

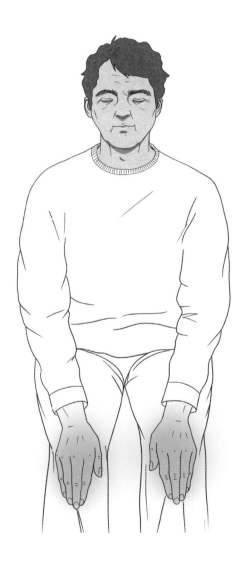

Feet

1. Hold one foot with both hands, with one hand on top of your foot and the other at the sole of your foot. You might be inclined to gently massage the soles of your feet. Repeat on the other foot.

2. Place your right hand on your right sole and your left hand on your left sole.

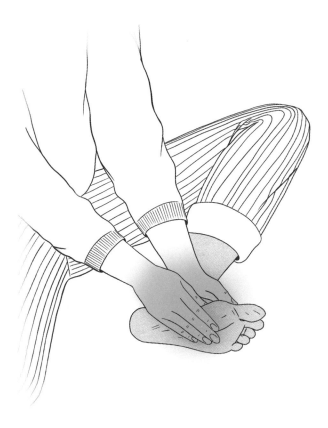

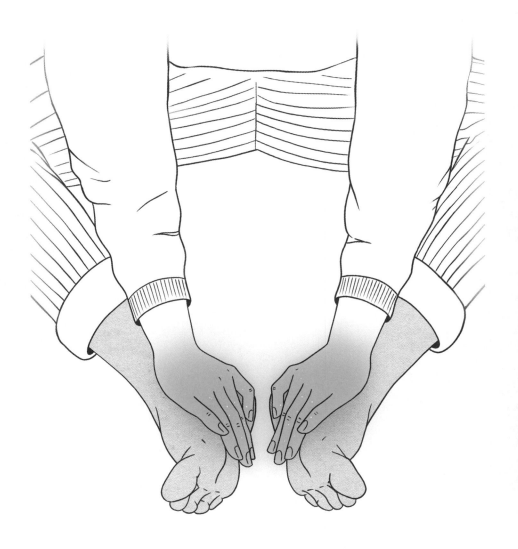

CHAPTER THREE

Reiki Symbols

During second-degree and third-degree Reiki training, the Reiki Master holds space for the attunement or placement process, where the practitioner is introduced to the symbols to help them evoke and connect to the Reiki energy. In the Usui system, there are four main symbols:

- Cho Ku Rei (Power Symbol)
- Sei Hei Ki (Mental/Emotional Symbol)
- Hon Sha Ze Sho Nen (Distant Symbol)
- Dai Ko Myo (Master Symbol)

If the symbols from your lineage differ from the ones in this book, I recommend sticking to the symbols your teacher introduced to you. Many versions of the symbols have been adapted and taught over the years, so you might see some variations based on the lineage. Remember, the intention when invoking the symbol is much more important than how the symbol looks. It is your intent that gives energy and power to these symbols.

This chapter discusses the use of these symbols, how to activate and draw them, and the pronunciations for each.

Activating the Symbols

There is no one way to activate the symbols. Experiment with various methods, and see what feels natural to you. Remember, the most important element is your intent. Here are a few ways to invoke the symbol:

1. Say the name of the symbol in your head or out loud three times.

2. Draw the symbol on your palms before placing your hands on the recipient.

3. Draw the symbol in the air above the recipient's body.

4. Visualize the symbol in your head.

NOTE: Always draw the strokes from left to right and top to bottom.

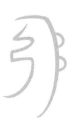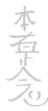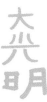

Cho Ku Rei (Power Symbol)

The first symbol, also known as the Power Symbol, is Cho Ku Rei (pronounced *cho ku ray*). Cho Ku Rei comes from Shintoism and means "by decree of the Divine." This symbol is generally used to protect and bless people and objects. You can use the Power Symbol anytime during the treatment, but it is especially powerful and effective when used at the beginning and end.

USES:

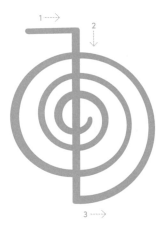

- Increases the strength of Reiki

- Seals and cleanses space around a recipient

- Clears negative energy

- Protects individuals and any object of value

- Protects individuals from psychic attack

- Heals physical pain

Sei Hei Ki (Mental/Emotional Symbol)

The second symbol, also known as the Mental/Emotional Symbol, is Sei Hei Ki (pronounced *say hay ki*). Sei Hei Ki is a Sanskrit seed syllable called *hrih*, which translates to "one's natural disposition."

Positive affirmations are more powerful when paired up with this symbol and can be incorporated into the treatment to release old, unwanted patterns and healing emotions.

USES:

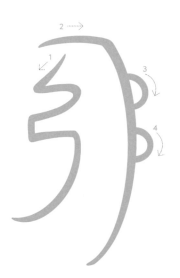

- Helps with overcoming addictions and releasing old, unwanted patterns

- Improves memory

- Enhances the use of affirmations

- Harmonizes both brain hemispheres to promote a sense of balance

- Empowers the heart and relationships

- Heals feelings and emotions

Hon Sha Ze Sho Nen (Distant Symbol)

The third symbol, also known as the Distant Symbol, is Hon Sha Ze Sho Nen (pronounced *hahn sha zey sho nen*). Hon Sha Ze Sho Nen translates to "the origin of all is pure consciousness" (a place where energy is not bound to time and space) in Japanese kanji. Consider this symbol a time machine or a bridge between different times and distances.

Invoke this symbol when you want to send healing to people you are not physically with as well as when you want to send healing to past and future events. If you are unsure of where to place your hands, Hon Sha Ze Sho Nen can also be used as a homing device during treatments, guiding the energy to flow where the recipient needs it the most.

USES:

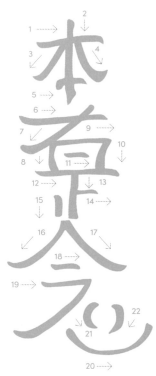

- Sends healing to people at a distance

- Sends healing to past and future events

- Empowers future goals

- Acts as a link to Source and higher consciousness

- Sends Reiki to the cause of the problem during treatments

- Aids in the release of unwanted, negative energies

Dai Ko Myo (Master Symbol)

The fourth symbol, also known as the Master Symbol, is Dai Ko Myo (pronounced *die ko mio*). This is the symbol given to Reiki practitioners attaining the Master level. It translates to "treasure house of the great beaming light" in Japanese and has the highest vibration among all Reiki symbols. Practitioners have reported that Dai Ko Myo feels very similar to Cho Ku Rei, except that it has a higher frequency, lasts longer, and acts as a stronger bridge between the practitioner and the source of Reiki. You can combine Dai Ko Myo with any of the other Usui Reiki symbols to increase its effectiveness.

USES:

- Strengthens connection to the higher self

- Heals a person's soul

- Helps one feel whole and fulfilled

- Blesses and empowers goals

- Strengthens the power of other symbols when used in conjunction

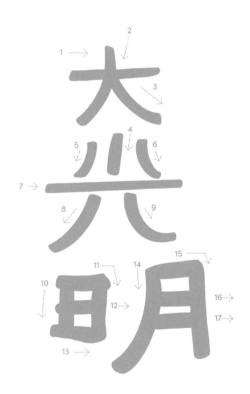

Symbol	Name and Pronunciation	Abbreviation	Alternative Name
	Cho Ku Rei *cho ku ray*	CKR	Power Symbol
	Sei Hei Ki *say hay ki*	SHK	Mental/ Emotional Symbol
	Hon Sha Ze Sho Nen *hahn sha zey sho nen*	HSZSN	Distant Symbol
	Dai Ko Myo *die ko mio*	DKM	Master Symbol

PART II

Treatment Sequences

The treatment sequences in this part are grouped into two categories: (1) common physical issues and concerns and (2) emotional, mental, and spiritual issues and concerns. Within those categories, the issues and concerns are arranged alphabetically for easy reference. The Appendix on page 184 offers a helpful illustration showing the location of major organs such as the kidneys, stomach, intestines, and more. I recommend using the information in this part of the book as a guide and starting point only; always rely on your intuition during your Reiki treatments.

About the Sequences

Here are several helpful points to keep in mind as you read the next chapters:

- See Chapter 2 for hand position guidance. The hand positions in these treatment sequences are derived from a melding of Dr. Usui's original hand positions, the Hayashi Healing Guide found in *Reiki: The Healing Touch: Japanese Reiki Techniques and Hayashi Healing Guide* by William Lee Rand, and my own experience. If there is a hand position or an area you feel guided to include that is not listed, honor your inner guidance. If you are unsure where exactly to place your hands, you can always invoke the Distant Symbol (Hon Sha Ze Sho Nen), as it can help Reiki travel to parts of the body where it's the most needed.

- To help with hand placement, an illustration of a human figure with numbered points of light is provided for each sequence. Each number corresponds to a matching step in the treatment sequence. For sequences that reference "affected areas," examples of affected areas are provided.

- The length of the treatment is up to you. I recommend spending at least three minutes on each position and preferably longer if you have the time.

- There is no wrong or right symbol to use for the various health issues. During treatment, notice which symbol(s) you feel most drawn and connected to. You can invoke the symbol(s) before you start the treatment by either drawing the symbol in the air or on your palms or saying the name of the symbol three times. Feel free to invoke the symbol throughout the session as many times as needed.

- For some of the emotional, mental, and spiritual issues, visualization meditations can help release energetic weight and give you further insight on what needs to be done to heal the issue. If you are treating yourself, record yourself saying the script (or your own version of it) and listen to it during self-treatment. If you are treating someone else, you can say it out loud in real time and guide the recipient through a visualization meditation either before or during the treatment.

- Thoughts and beliefs can speed up or hinder the healing process. Positive affirmations can help the recipient acknowledge their limiting beliefs and overcome self-sabotage. For those treatment sequences that include an affirmation, the recipient should say the affirmation out loud three times during the treatment; encourage them to do so with confidence and authority. You can also create your own positive affirmations for yourself and/or your recipients. Writing the affirmation down and posting it where it can be seen daily helps drive home the message.

Important note: Reiki is not meant to replace medical treatments or be used as a substitute for a physician's or therapist's care. For more serious illnesses, a specialist should always be consulted. Reiki can be used as a form of preventive medicine and as a complement to conventional treatments. Reiki is especially helpful during the recovery process because it helps the body return to homeostasis, which then speeds up the body's ability to heal. Reiki can also be used to help manage the anxiety and stress that accompany pain and suffering.

CHAPTER FOUR

Common Physical Issues and Concerns

The entries in this section are some of the most common physical issues and concerns for which Reiki has been helpful in speeding up the healing and recovery process. Refer to the following illustration of human anatomy and the female reproductive system as needed.

Acne

Generally, acne signals some sort of imbalance in the body. Reiki can help by bringing the body back into balance. Do not place your hands directly on the affected areas; rather, beam a few inches above.

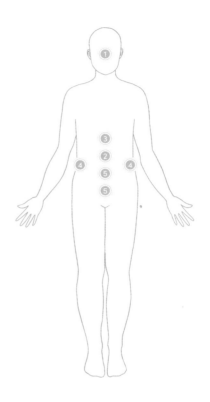

1. Affected areas (for example, face)
2. Liver
3. Stomach
4. Kidneys
5. Large intestine and small intestine

TIP: While it is helpful to think and meditate on the cause of acne, a dermatologist or aesthetician should be consulted to determine the cause of the problem.

Anemia

Anemia is a condition in which the body is lacking sufficient healthy red blood cells. Reiki can assist in the relief of associated symptoms—from fatigue and shortness of breath to dizziness and skin pallor.

1. Top of the head
2. Back of the head
3. Forehead
4. Temples
5. Back of the neck
6. Throat
7. Heart
8. Stomach
9. Palms of the hands
10. Soles of the feet

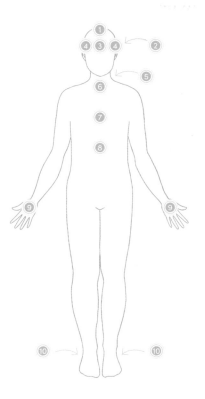

Ankle Pain

Ankle pain may occur from
an injury, overuse, or arthritis.
Regardless of the cause, Reiki is
an excellent complement to other
therapies intended to heal and/or
soothe painful muscles, joints, and
tendons.

1. One hand on the outer
   side of the ankle and one
   hand on the inner side of
   the ankle. (Repeat on the
   other side.)
2. Hands wrapped around
   each ankle at the
   same time.

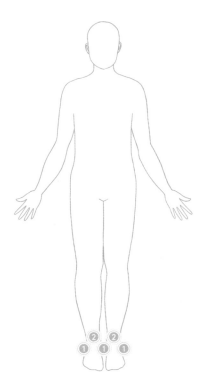

Aphasia and Other Speech Disorders

The inability to verbally express oneself clearly can be frustrating. Although some speech disorders cannot be cured, Reiki can help relieve frustration and remove obstacles in the way of reaching one's realistic communication goals.

1. Forehead
2. Temples
3. Top of the throat

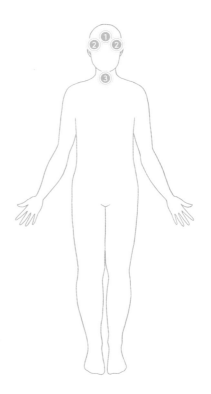

Appendectomy Recovery

An appendectomy is an emergency surgery to remove an infected appendix. Reiki can support the recovery process, which may take anywhere from one to four weeks.

1. Top of the head
2. Back of the head
3. Temples
4. Forehead
5. Appendix
6. Stomach

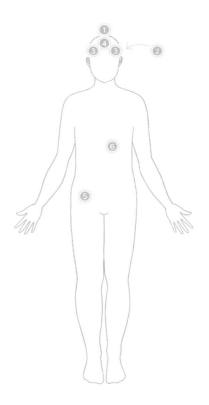

Arthritis

Arthritis is a long-term condition that often relies heavily on medical pain management. Reiki can be an important complement to the traditional approach to help the recipient further manage their pain.

1. Affected joints
   (for example, hands)

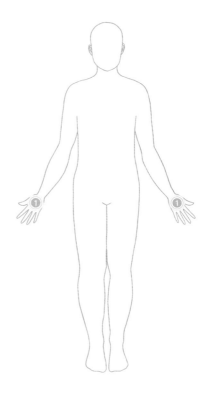

Asthma

People with asthma typically need an inhaler in emergency situations, but when they are looking for some support to facilitate deeper breaths and calm the nerves in general, Reiki is an excellent choice.

1. Forehead
2. Sides of the nose
3. Throat
4. Heart
5. Beneath the sternum

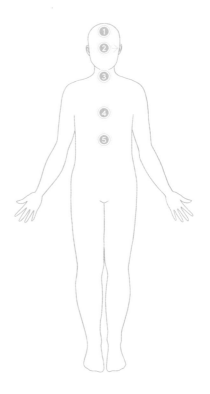

Back Pain

Chronic back pain can interfere with every aspect of life, usually making pain management a priority. Although Reiki cannot replace medical intervention, it is helpful for relaxing tense areas, thereby providing pain relief.

1. Lower back (on stomach)
2. Middle back (on stomach)
3. Along the spine (on stomach)

TIP: For self-treatment, sit up on a comfortable chair or mattress.

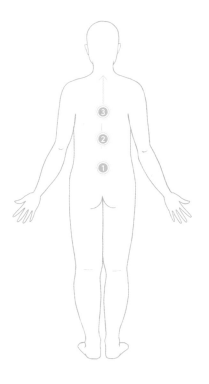

Broken Bones

After a broken bone has been reset, sending Reiki to the area may assist with the bone knitting process. Use your best judgment to decide whether you should place your hands directly on the affected area or beam a few inches above.

1. Affected area (for example, right wrist)

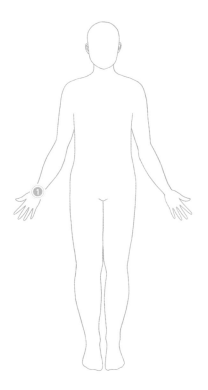

Bronchitis

Coughing up mucus and shortness of breath are hallmarks of bronchitis. This can be very stressful on the mind and body, so sending Reiki to the affected areas can offer much-needed relief.

1. Bronchial tubes
2. Over the throat
3. Chest
4. Heart

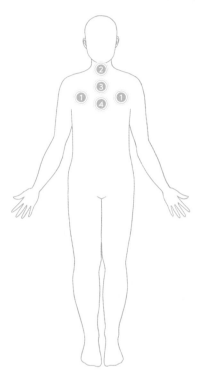

Bruises

No one is a stranger to the occasional bruise, so you may find your hands guided to them, either on yourself or others, to offer some Reiki healing. Use your best judgment to determine whether you should place your hands directly on the affected area or beam a few inches above.

1. Affected area
   (for example, left shin)

TIP: For fresh bruises, an immediate application of ice can reduce the amount of blood that pools under the skin. Arnica gel or cream can help facilitate blood flow and reabsorb bruising.

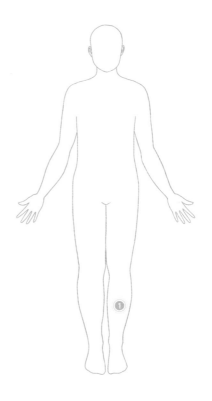

Cancer

While Reiki should never replace a patient's regular cancer treatment, it can bring comfort, balance, and relaxation to patients who are undergoing chemotherapy.

1. Affected area(s)/location of tumor(s) (for example, breasts)

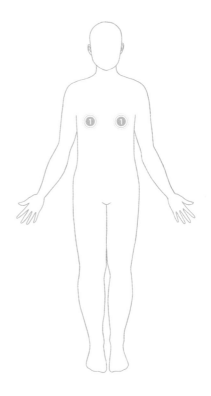

Cold Sores

The herpes simplex virus, which causes cold sores, can be activated during times of stress or fatigue and when the immune system is weak. Lengthy sun exposure and extreme temperatures can also be culprits. Do not place your hands directly on the affected area; beam a few inches above.

1. Affected area
   (for example, lips)

TIP: Cold sores are often one of the first signs that more sleep and rest are needed.

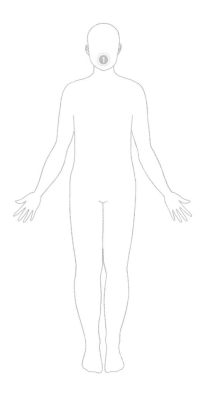

Colds

The common cold is a condition that usually needs to run its course; while waiting for it to resolve, Reiki can offer symptom relief.

1. Over the throat
2. Lungs
3. Back of the neck
4. Chest

TIP: At the first symptoms of a cold, dress warmly and cover the chest, even indoors. Outside, cover the back of the neck with a scarf. Echinacea, elderberry, vitamin C, and zinc are some immune-boosting supplements to consider.

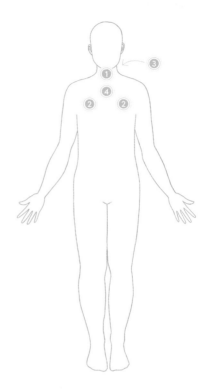

Cough

Whether it's a dry cough or one that brings up a lot of mucus, coughing can have a negative effect on the body. Reiki is an excellent complement to over-the-counter medicine as well as home remedies for relieving coughs (see the tip below).

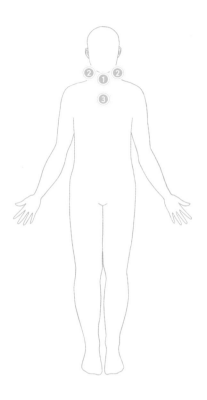

1. Over the throat
2. Sides of the neck
3. Chest

TIP: To soothe a cough, apply a heating pad over the chest for about 10 to 20 minutes. Steamy, hot showers or baths can also help soothe a cough and clear up the mucus.

Diabetes

Put simply, diabetes is a condition in which the body has difficulty processing sugar. Although medical intervention and dietary changes are essential for management, Reiki can offer further improvements.

1. Top of the head
2. Back of the head
3. Forehead
4. Temples
5. Heart
6. Liver
7. Pancreas
8. Stomach
9. Bladder area

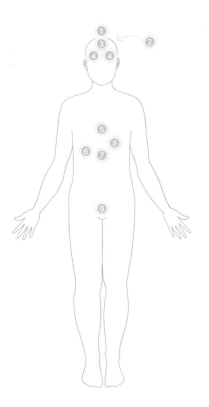

Digestive Complaints

Eating whole foods high in fiber mindfully and slowly can aid digestion, but sometimes, digestive complaints arise seemingly for no reason. Whatever imbalance is causing the discomfort, Reiki can help the body regain homeostasis.

1. Over the mouth
2. Liver
3. Stomach
4. Large and small intestine

TIP: Spend time sending Reiki to the food you plan to eat: hold your hands a few inches above the food for about two minutes or longer if you feel guided to do so. Set your intention for the food to be well digested by the body.

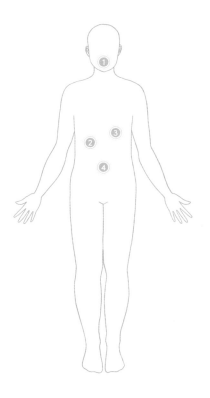

Dislocated Joints

Even after a dislocated joint has been properly popped back into place, the associated pain tends to linger. Enter Reiki. Use your best judgment to see if you should place your hands directly on the affected area or beam a few inches above.

1. Affected area
   (for example, right shoulder)

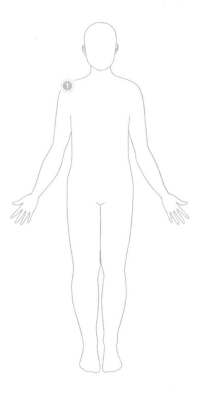

Dizziness

There are numerous causes of frequent dizziness, each requiring a different treatment. Once serious issues have been ruled out or treated, Reiki can help the body regain its equilibrium.

1. Top of the head
2. Back of the head
3. Forehead
4. Temples
5. Heart

TIP: The recipient should drink plenty of water both before and after the Reiki treatment.

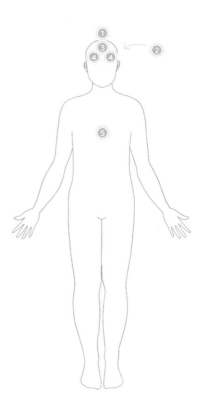

Ear Pain

Whether ear pain is caused by an ear infection, high altitudes, or something else, Reiki can have a soothing effect on this condition.

1. Cupped hands placed over each ear
2. Index fingers placed in the back lower pocket of the ears, letting the middle and ring fingers rest on top of the ears

TIP: Wet a few paper towels with water and microwave for about 20 seconds. Squeeze most of the water out, place the paper towels in a paper cup, and hold the opening of the cup over the ear for a few minutes. Repeat for the other side.

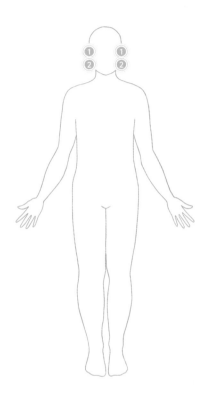

Fatigue

Fatigue can be a consequence of a busy life as well as an indication of something more serious. Whether fatigue is a result of an overactive lifestyle or a symptom of another condition, Reiki can help replenish and sustain one's body energy reserves. Following treatment, do the "Visualization Meditation for Fatigue" on page 115.

1. Top of the head
2. Back of the head
3. Forehead
4. Cupped hands placed gently over the eyes
5. Heart chakra

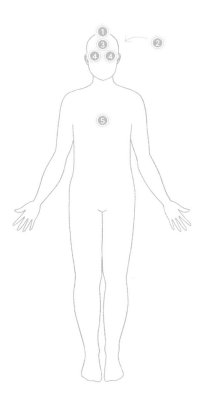

TIP: Power naps of 30 minutes or less can work wonders during the day.

VISUALIZATION MEDITATION FOR FATIGUE

1. Sit down and bring your hands to your heart center in Gassho meditation.

2. Gently close your eyes and imagine that the top of your head is wide open like a door.

3. Imagine this white or golden light pouring in from the sky, from Source, entering your head and filling every inch of your being all the way down to your fingertips and toes.

4. Imagine this healing, soothing light filling in every crevasse, every gap, and every crack of your body.

5. Allow this light to enter, fill you up, energize you, and nourish every inch of your being.

6. Continue to meditate for 15 minutes or more.

Fever

When the body is trying to fight an infection or an illness, body temperature often increases, resulting in a fever. In addition to mainstream treatments, Reiki can assist in bringing body temperature closer to a normal level.

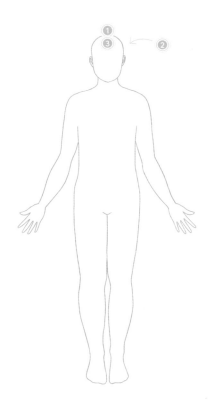

1. Top of the head
2. Back of the head
3. Forehead

TIP: It is important to stay hydrated when body temperature is high. Water, coconut water, ice chips, herbal teas, bone broth, and ice pops are all great options.

Flu

Being sick in bed with the flu is not fun, and even after the flu has run its course, the body may feel weak and depleted. In addition to rest, sleep, and naps (as needed), a Reiki session can help the body bounce back more quickly after the ordeal.

1. Top of the head
2. Back of the head
3. Forehead
4. Temples
5. Heart
6. Lungs
7. Stomach

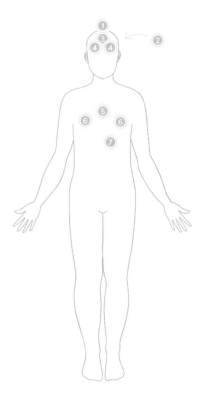

Food Poisoning

A bout of food poisoning causes vomiting and diarrhea and usually lasts a day or so. While it passes relatively quickly, it's not uncommon to feel a little beat up afterward. A Reiki session can help the digestive system recover more fully.

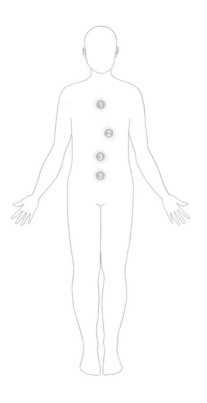

1. Chest
2. Stomach
3. Large intestine and small intestine

TIP: Be gentle on the digestive system following a bout of food poisoning; the BRAT diet (bananas, rice, applesauce, and toast) is a good choice. Also, it is advised to drink water with electrolytes to replenish lost minerals.

Gallstones

Gallstones cause a gnawing discomfort or sharp pain in the body and often need to be removed surgically. This is a painful condition for which Reiki can offer some relief.

1. Liver
2. Stomach
3. Large intestine and small intestine

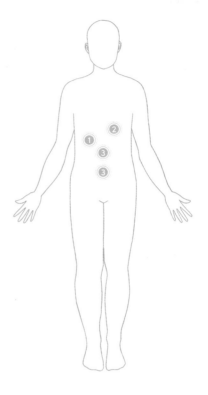

Gastritis

Gastritis is inflammation in the lin-
ing of the stomach and can have a
variety of causes. It isn't necessary
to know the cause to soothe the
inflammation with a Reiki session in concert with any necessary
medical and alternative remedies.

1. Top of the head
2. Back of the head
3. Forehead
4. Temples
5. Beneath the sternum
6. Stomach
7. Large and small intestine

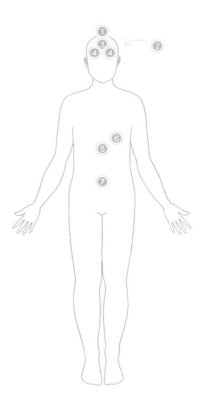

Hair Loss

Whether male or female, hair loss is concerning to most and may cause feelings of embarrassment and sadness. Regardless of the reason for the hair loss (for example, male pattern baldness or chemotherapy), Reiki has its place as a complementary treatment.

1. Top of the head
2. Back of the head
3. Forehead
4. Temples
5. Stomach
6. Large intestine and small intestine

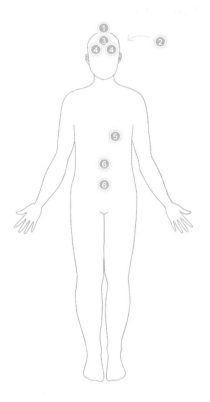

Headache

Headaches, which have a variety of causative factors, are quite common. Beaming Reiki to the head gives the blood vessels and nerves responsible for the pain a chance to relax and can be very comforting to the recipient.

1. Top of the head
2. Back of the head
3. Forehead
4. Temples

TIP: Spend most of the session placing your hands on the area of the head that aches. Experiment with the pressure of your hands. Sometimes switching off between holding the head tightly and letting go of some pressure back and forth helps relieve some tension in the head.

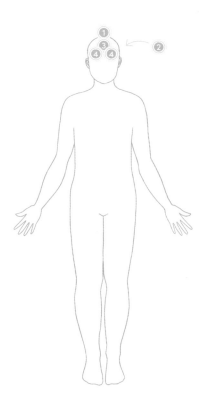

Heatstroke

Heatstroke is a medical emergency that requires immediate intervention. With confusion, slurred speech, and delirium as potential symptoms, it's quite frightening to experience. Following treatment, Reiki can help the mind resolve lingering fears.

1. Top of the head
2. Back of the head
3. Forehead
4. Temples
5. Lungs
6. Chest
7. Heart
8. Stomach
9. Large intestine and small intestine

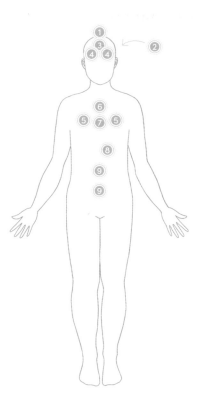

Hernia

A hernia is an organ or fatty tissue that bulges through a weak spot in muscle or tissue. This causes pain and discomfort, which is where Reiki can help the most. Medical intervention is usually required to repair the hernia.

1. Stomach
2. Large intestine and small intestine

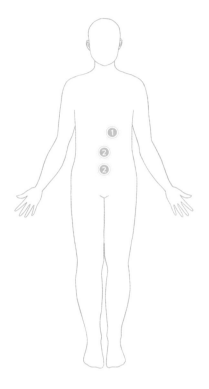

Hiccups

Who hasn't had a bout of hiccups? They usually go away on their own, but when they don't, there may be an underlying cause that should be checked out. If more serious issues have been ruled out, Reiki is an excellent choice for relief.

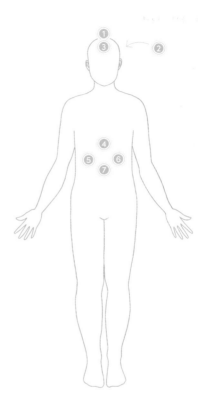

1. Top of the head
2. Back of the head
3. Forehead
4. Diaphragm
5. Liver
6. Stomach
7. Pancreas

TIP: While there are many remedies to relieve hiccups, here are two that I've found helpful: (1) Hold your breath and swallow your spit three times, or (2) suck on a teaspoon of sugar until the hiccups stop.

High Blood Pressure

High blood pressure is a common condition that requires monitoring by a healthcare practitioner. When blood pressure is properly controlled, Reiki is an excellent adjunct for keeping levels stable through relaxation.

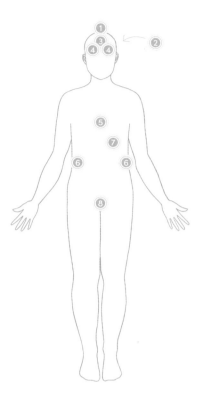

1. Top of the head
2. Back of the head
3. Forehead
4. Temples
5. Heart
6. Kidneys
7. Stomach
8. Bladder area

Insomnia

Possible causes of insomnia include stress, anxiety, depression, inconsistent sleep schedule, physical injuries, and specific sleep disorders. It is worthwhile to determine the cause of the restlessness and work on healing the issue with Reiki's assistance.

1. Crown chakra
2. Temples
3. Cupped hands placed gently over the eyes
4. Root chakra

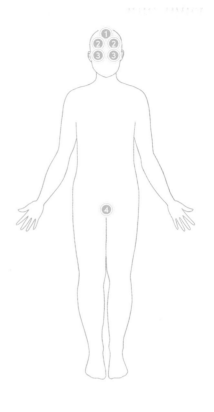

TIP: Blue-light blocking lightbulbs have warm, soft tones that support the body's natural melatonin production (a hormone necessary for a good night's sleep). Guided meditations specifically for sleeping are available on YouTube and meditation apps such as Calm. Technology aside, counting slowly from 100 to 1 while imagining melting into the mattress deeper and deeper with every exhale is a great technique.

Intestinal Parasites

Intestinal parasites come with a host of uncomfortable symptoms, including gas, bloating, stomach pain, and fatigue. Even after parasites are expelled from the body, it may take some time for the symptoms to resolve. In the meantime, Reiki can soothe the system.

1. Top of the head
2. Back of the head
3. Forehead
4. Temples
5. Stomach
6. Large intestine and small intestine

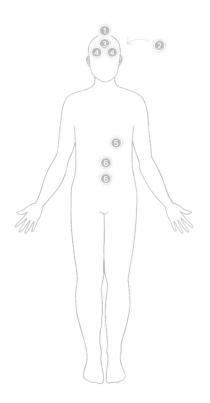

Knee Pain

Whether it's chronic or temporary, knee pain hinders the ability to enjoy physical activity. Assuming there are no serious issues, you can send Reiki directly to the knees to offer relief from the discomfort so that usual activities can soon be resumed.

1. One hand over the kneecap and the other hand under the kneecap
2. Repeat on the other side
3. Cupped hands placed atop each knee

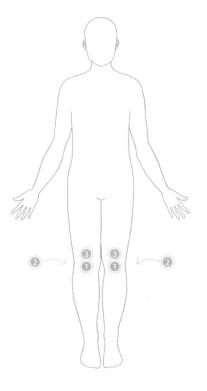

Measles

Measles is an infectious disease caused by a highly contagious virus. Therefore, Reiki should only be performed for others after the infection has been resolved. During recovery, Reiki can support the body's return to full health.

1. Top of the head
2. Back of the head
3. Forehead
4. Temples
5. Heart
6. Stomach
7. Large intestine and small intestine

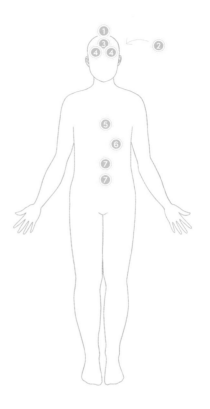

Menopause

Menopause is a naturally occur-
ring stage in many women's lives.
However, it is often accompanied
by uncomfortable symptoms. Reiki
can support this experience by
helping alleviate the unwanted
side effects of lower estro-
gen levels.

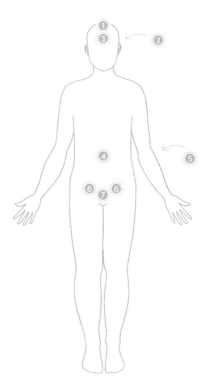

1. Top of the head
2. Back of the head
3. Forehead
4. Lower abdomen
5. Lower back
6. Ovaries on both sides
7. Uterus (womb)

Menstrual Cramps

Some people struggle with menstrual cramps every month for years on end. While several remedies and treatments are available to relieve the discomfort, sending Reiki to the areas of pain can feel supportive and nurturing, potentially reducing the pain or rendering it more tolerable.

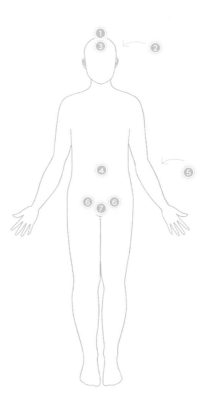

1. Top of the head
2. Back of the head
3. Forehead
4. Lower abdomen
5. Lower back
6. Ovaries on both sides
7. Uterus (womb)

TIP: Place a heating pad or a heated blanket over the area of pain for some relief.

Morning Sickness

During the first trimester, pregnant women commonly complain of morning sickness (which can occur at any time of day). For some, it lasts beyond the first trimester. Reiki is perfectly safe to perform during pregnancy and is very useful for settling the stomach.

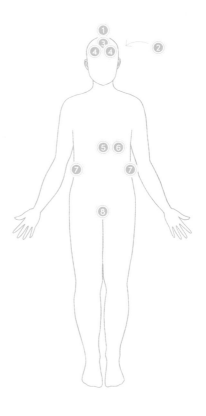

1. Top of the head
2. Back of the head
3. Forehead
4. Temples
5. Beneath the sternum
6. Stomach
7. Kidneys
8. Uterus

TIP: Drinking ginger tea can help reduce nausea during pregnancy.

Nausea

Feeling the need to vomit is among the most distress-ing symptoms of a variety of conditions—from eating something spoiled to motion sickness. When the feeling persists without vom-iting, Reiki can help relieve the distress.

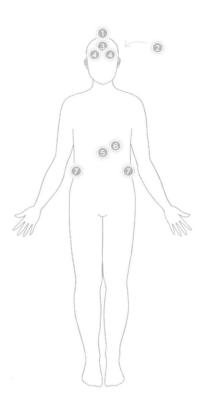

1. Top of the head
2. Back of the head
3. Forehead
4. Temples
5. Beneath the sternum
6. Stomach
7. Kidneys

TIP: Sucking on a ginger lozenge can help reduce nausea.

Night Terrors in Children

Although not all children experience them, night terrors (also known as sleep terrors) are a normal stage of childhood development. Even so, they are certainly undesired and frightening. A child who receives Reiki sessions may sleep better and have fewer of these occurrences.

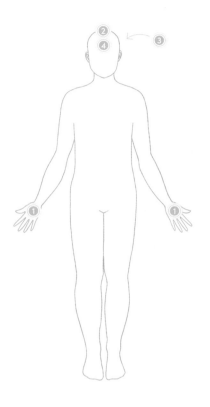

1. Palms of the hands
2. Top of the head
3. Back of the head
4. Forehead

TIP: For children who are prone to night terrors, it is helpful to turn on the lights so that the child knows that they are having a dream. Gently pat the child's back and soothe them with comforting words.

Nosebleed

The tiny blood vessels in the nose tend to bleed easily. Nosebleeds are often caused by dry climates or may be the result of a blow to the nose. Reiki can be beamed to the nose while getting the blood to stop flowing.

1. Place the thumb and index finger on the sides of the nose.
2. Hold the nostrils closed for 10 minutes or less while the recipient breathes through the mouth.

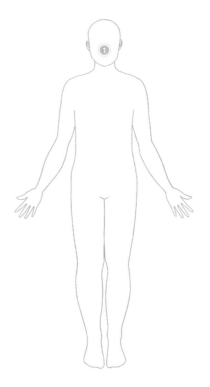

Obesity

Obesity is a condition in which a person has too much body fat. Aside from a host of physical symptoms, obesity often carries with it negative feelings about one's body. Reiki can help the recipient find love and appreciation for their body while they take steps to aim for a healthier state of being.

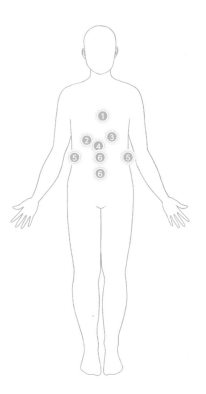

1. Heart
2. Liver
3. Stomach
4. Pancreas
5. Kidneys
6. Large intestine and small intestine

Pregnancy

It's completely safe and healthy to practice Reiki on pregnant women, as Reiki will have a calming and healing effect on the mother, which will also positively affect the baby. Reiki is also known to help mothers feel at peace with the physical, emotional, and mental shifts that come with pregnancy and feel more connected to their baby spiritually.

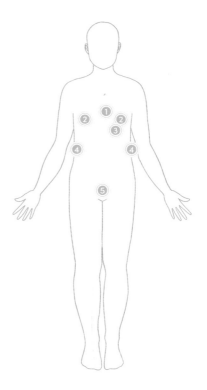

1. Heart
2. Breasts
3. Stomach
4. Sides of the waist
5. Uterus (womb)

Scarlet Fever

Scarlet fever is a bacterial infection that usually causes a bright red rash over much of the body, along with high fever and a sore throat. It requires antibiotics to resolve. Once the infection is no longer contagious, Reiki can help the body return to homeostasis.

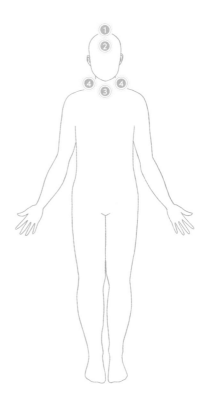

1. Top of the head
2. Forehead
3. Over the throat
4. Sides of the throat
5. Hands placed a few inches over areas of rash

Seasickness

Seasickness is a type of motion sickness that occurs during travel over water. When there's no immediate chance of getting to solid ground, Reiki can offer relief of cold sweats, dizziness, and nausea.

1. Stomach
2. Top of the head
3. Back of the head
4. Forehead
5. Temples

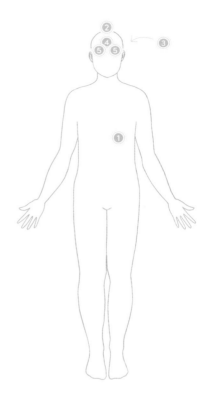

Shoulder Pain

Persistent shoulder pain may require a trip inside an MRI machine to determine the source of the problem. Reiki can help the recipient find relief from the associated inflammation and discomfort of a damaged muscle, tendon, or ligament.

1. Shoulders
2. Back of the neck

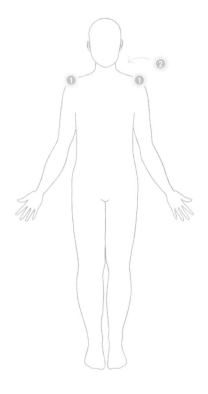

Skin Rash

A rash can be the side effect of infections, allergens, medical disorders, and medications, among other causes. While the underlying cause is being treated, Reiki can support the body's healing processes. Use your best judgment to see if you should place your hands directly on the affected area or beam a few inches above.

1. Affected area
   (for example, chest)

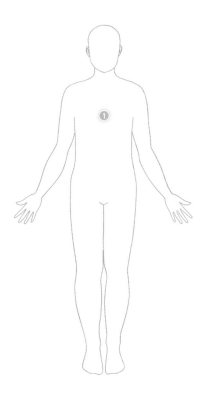

Sore Throat

A sore throat is not only uncomfortable but also a likely sign that the body is fighting off a virus. A strong immune system is essential to fend off the invader. Reiki can act as an immune system booster, along with other remedies (see tip below).

1. Over the throat area
2. Sides of the throat
3. Back of the neck

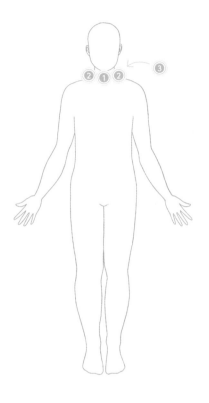

TIP: At the first symptoms of a sore throat, it's advised to drink a lot of warm tea with honey. Ginger, licorice root, marshmallow root, and green tea are great options. Gargling for about 10 seconds three times a day with a half cup of warm water mixed with a half teaspoon of salt helps draw out any virus and bacteria in the throat.

Splinters

When a foreign body sticks into the skin, it must come out, but it's not always so easy. Reiki can bring calm around the inevitable poking and prodding. Use your best judgment to see if you should place your hands directly on the affected area or beam a few inches above.

1. Affected area
    (for example, left ring finger)

TIP: Pour a tablespoon of hydrogen peroxide over the affected area and then use a clean pair of tweezers to pick the splinter out.

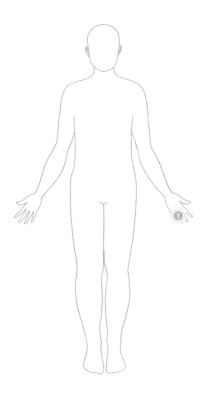

Stomach Pain

A bellyache is one of those ail-
ments we all experience from time
to time, usually the result of a little
excess gas because of something
we've eaten. Sending Reiki to the
belly does wonders for relaxing
the muscles and relieving the gas.

1. Beneath the ribs
2. Stomach
3. Lower belly

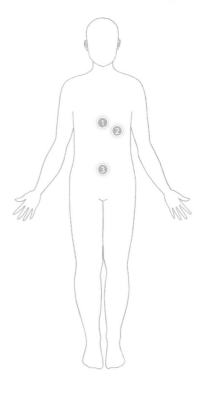

Tinnitus
(Ringing in the Ear)

Ringing in the ears is a persistent complaint for some people and has a variety of causes, though for the majority it is a temporary condition that often results from loud sounds. Reiki can be comforting when beamed to the ears, potentially relaxing the tiny bones, cartilage, and hairs.

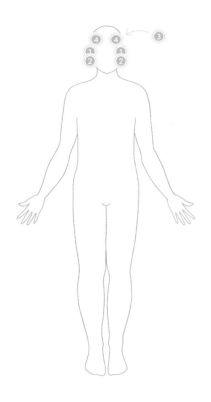

1. Cupped hands placed over each ear
2. Index fingers placed in the back lower pocket of the ears and with the middle and ring fingers resting on top of the ears
3. Back of the head
4. Temples

Toothache

First stop: dentist. Second stop: Reiki practitioner. As much as a dentist might do to relieve a toothache, including pulling out the affected tooth or performing a root canal, the pain often lingers and additional support is needed.

1. Affected area from outside the mouth (for example, front tooth)
2. Sides of the jaw

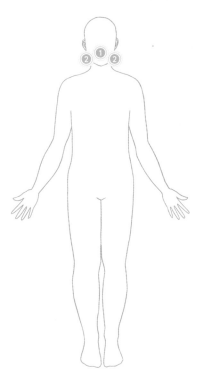

Tonsillitis

The tonsils are tissues on either side of the back of the throat. As the name implies, tonsillitis is inflammation of those tissues. Sometimes they need to be surgically removed, but not always. Either way, Reiki treatment can provide much-needed pain relief.

1. Over the throat

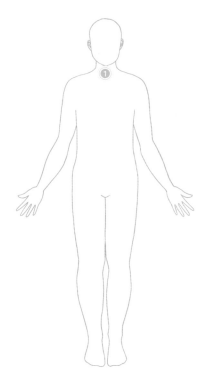

Urinary Tract Infection (UTI)

An infection in the urinary tract can be quite uncomfortable. Reiki can support the body in the healing process, but steps should be taken to resolve the issue so that the condition doesn't become more serious (see tip below).

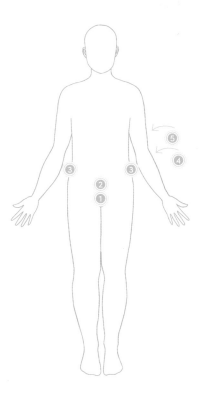

1. Uterus, if applicable
2. Bladder
3. Kidneys
4. Lower back
5. Side back (both sides)

TIP: At the first symptoms of a UTI, it is advised to drink plenty of water, increase vitamin C intake, and avoid sexual intercourse until symptom-free. If symptoms worsen over time, a doctor should be consulted; antibiotics are an effective treatment for UTIs and can stop bacteria from traveling to the kidneys, which could result in a kidney infection.

Vision Problems

Vision problems run the gamut from simple nearsightedness and farsightedness to more serious issues like glaucoma and macular degeneration. Beaming Reiki to the eyes sends healing energy to these essential tools for navigating the world.

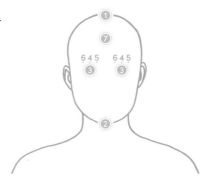

1. Top of the head
2. Bottom of the head
3. Cupped hands placed gently over the eyes
4. Place index, middle, and ring fingers over each eyelid with very little pressure
5. Place index fingers gently on the inside corners of the eyes
6. Place index fingers gently on the outside corners of the eyes
7. Third eye chakra (the point in middle of the eyebrows)

Vomiting

Vomiting is often necessary after something toxic or spoiled has been ingested. The aim is not to stop the vomiting with Reiki but to help the body recover from the experience.

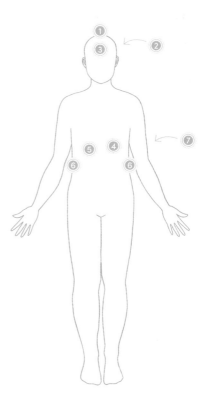

1. Top of the head
2. Back of the head
3. Forehead
4. Stomach
5. Liver
6. Kidneys
7. Along the spine

Whooping Cough

This respiratory infection is highly contagious and requires medical intervention. Reiki should only be performed for others to help the body return to homeostasis after the infection has been cleared.

1. Top of the head
2. Back of the head
3. Forehead
4. Temples
5. Throat
6. Lungs
7. Heart
8. Beneath the sternum
9. Stomach
10. Large intestine and small intestine

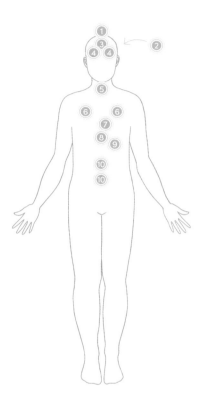

Wounds

Whether slicing one's hand while cutting produce, tripping and scraping a knee, or cutting one's forehead on an open cabinet door, people are bound to have accidents resulting in wounds. Once the area has been cleansed and treated, Reiki can help ease the pain and promote healing. Use your best judgment to determine whether you should place your hands directly on the affected area or beam a few inches above.

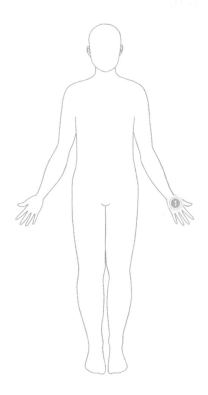

1. Affected area
   (for example, left hand)

CHAPTER FIVE

Mental, Emotional, and Spiritual Issues and Concerns

Mental, emotional, and spiritual issues and concerns have multiple causes. Talk therapy with a therapist and/or guidance from a trusted spiritual adviser paired with Reiki can speed up the healing process and help us gain a better understanding of our multidimensional self and how we have been navigating the world. In this section, you will find treatment sequences for some of the most common mental, emotional, and spiritual issues and concerns for which people seek Reiki.

Note: If you ever feel that your mental health is at risk, seek a licensed therapist for help and encourage others to do the same.

Anger

Anger is a natural response to an injustice or a threat and serves an important purpose. Unresolved and repressed anger, however, can negatively affect the body and mind. Reiki can provide people with insight into where the anger stems from and process it in a healthy way.

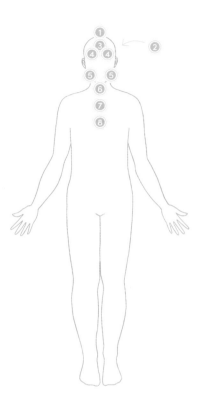

1. Top of the head
2. Back of the head
3. Forehead
4. Temples
5. Sides of the jaw
6. Throat chakra
7. Chest
8. Heart chakra

Anxiety

Anxiety that interferes with daily functioning should be discussed with a healthcare professional. Reiki can support the body in relieving the uncomfortable symptoms that often accompany this condition as well as soothe the mind. The 4-7-8 breathing technique on page 34 should be performed prior to treatment for grounding as many times as needed until relaxation is achieved.

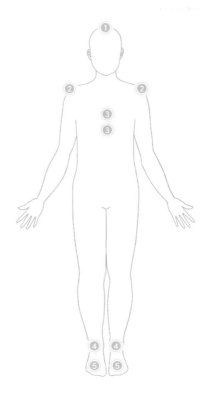

1. Crown chakra
2. Shoulders
3. Heart chakra and solar plexus chakra (one hand on each)
4. Ankles
5. Soles of the feet

TIP: During step three, guide the recipient to connect to the rhythm of their breath, noticing the rise and fall of their stomach while focusing on their breath and the present moment.

AFFIRMATION

I am here now.

Authentic Self

The authentic self is who we truly are deep down. Reiki can help this part of our being emerge and therefore build a life that aligns with our core values and identities. Invoke the Master Symbol (Dai Ko Myo) anytime you feel inclined throughout the treatment.

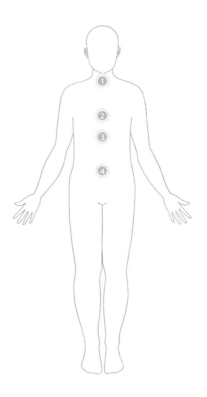

1. Throat chakra
2. Heart chakra
3. Solar plexus chakra
4. Sacral chakra

AFFIRMATION

When I am being my true self, I feel at ease. I am loved just as I am.

Concentration

When the mind is scattered with thoughts, it's hard to concentrate on the task at hand. Reiki aids concentration by relaxing the mind and improving mental focus. Invoke the Mental/Emotional Symbol (Sei Hei Ki) anytime you feel inclined throughout the treatment.

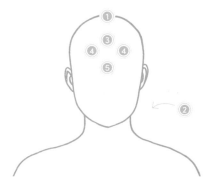

1. Top of the head
2. Back of the head
3. Forehead
4. Temples
5. Third eye chakra

AFFIRMATION

I have clarity and energy. I free myself from distractions.

Creativity

When creativity feels elusive, Reiki can help clear energetic obstacles that may be blocking the way to creative manifestation and bring in new inspiration.

1. Third eye chakra
2. Throat chakra
3. Sacral chakra

AFFIRMATION

I release all resistance to expressing my creativity fully.

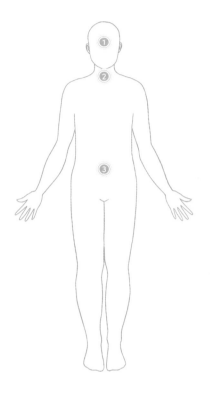

Depression

Persistent feelings of sadness, apathy, or suicidal thoughts require immediate consultation with a mental health specialist. However, feeling depressed or sad from time to time is a normal human condition. Reiki can be comforting to the mind and body during this time and help strengthen the connection to Source, alleviating the melancholy.

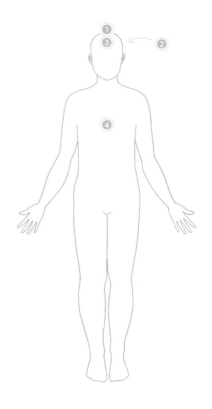

1. Top of the head
2. Back of the head
3. Forehead
4. Heart chakra

TIP: While receiving Reiki for depression, the recipient should touch the tip of the index finger to the thumb while keeping the other three fingers relaxed.

AFFIRMATION

I am not my emotions or my thoughts. When I am feeling depressed, I show myself kindness and forgiveness.

Divine Connection

A Reiki session allows the mind and body to fully relax into the moment, enabling space for divine connection to shine through.

1. Crown chakra
2. Third eye chakra
3. Gassho meditation

AFFIRMATION

I am always guided, protected, and loved. I am truly never alone.

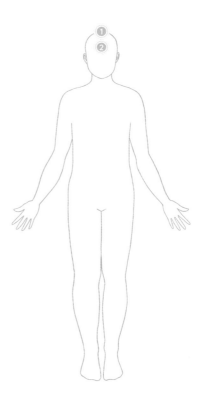

Forgiveness for Others

Holding on to anger serves no one. With intention, a Reiki session can help the recipient connect with their inner compassion and forgiveness, often even in grievous circumstances. See the "The Ho'oponopono Prayer" on page 164 for further assistance. Invoke the Mental/Emotional Symbol (Sei Hei Ki) anytime you feel inclined throughout the treatment.

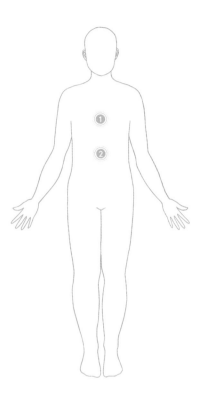

1. Heart chakra
2. Solar plexus chakra

AFFIRMATION

I release the pain of anger and rage from my body. I accept my past and learn from it.

THE HO'OPONOPONO PRAYER

This is a Hawaiian practice for forgiveness that I was taught by one of my Reiki Master teachers and have found very helpful in my life. Reciting the Ho'oponopono Prayer is a beautiful, effective method for forgiving and letting go of the anger toward someone who has hurt you.

The words of the prayer are: *"Please forgive me, I'm sorry, I love you and thank you."* Say the prayer out loud three times whenever you find yourself thinking about the person you want to forgive.

It might be difficult to muster compassion and send healing to someone who has hurt you, but as you heal and gain more clarity, you learn that their actions had less to do with you and more to do with them. You understand that they wouldn't have acted that way if they were whole and healed themselves. People who are hurting tend to hurt other people.

When you understand this, you can see them as a divine being, navigating through their own fears, trauma, stress, challenges, and obstacles every day, just like everyone else on this planet. Perceiving this person as being on their own spiritual journey brings compassion. That's the "I love you" part of this prayer. As for the "thank you," you are not thanking anyone for mistreating you but for being an active participant in your self-worth, growth, and healing.

Forgiveness for Self

We all do things we regret, but we deserve to forgive ourselves just as much as others deserve forgiveness. Reiki can bring emotional healing around past mistakes.

1. Heart chakra
2. Solar plexus chakra

AFFIRMATION

I am done beating myself up for what has happened in the past. I am learning and growing every day.

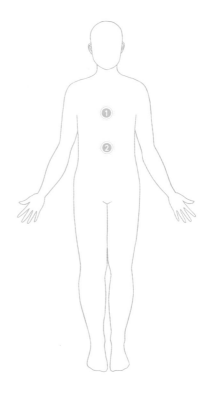

Goal Empowerment

Pursuing a goal sometimes feels scary or impossible. Reiki helps break down any self-limiting blocks that are obstructing what one sets out to achieve. For additional support, see "Visualizing the Outcome" to follow. Invoke the Master Symbol (Dai Ko Myo) and the Distant Symbol (Hon Sha Ze Sho Nen) anytime you feel inclined throughout the treatment.

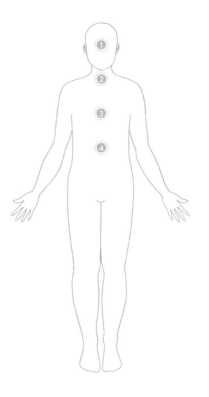

1. Third eye chakra
2. Throat chakra
3. Heart chakra
4. Solar plexus chakra

AFFIRMATION

I turn my dreams into goals, my goals into plans, and my plans into reality.

VISUALIZING THE OUTCOME

1. On a piece of paper, write your name, a description of your goal, and the Distant Symbol.

2. Fold the paper small enough to fit between your palms.

3. Spend about 15 minutes a day visualizing the desired outcome as you meditate with that piece of paper between your hands.

Tip: You can carry this piece of paper with you in your pocket and beam it Reiki throughout the day or whenever you think about your goals, or you can advise the recipient to do so.

Grief

With loss comes grief. The only way to work through the grief is to accept and feel the emotions as they arise. Reiki can help ease some of the most debilitating emotional pain during the grieving process. Invoke the Mental/Emotional Symbol (Sei Hei Ki) anytime you feel inclined throughout the treatment.

1. Crown chakra
2. Sides of the nose
3. Throat chakra
4. Lungs
5. Diaphragm
6. Ribs
7. Heart chakra
8. Root chakra

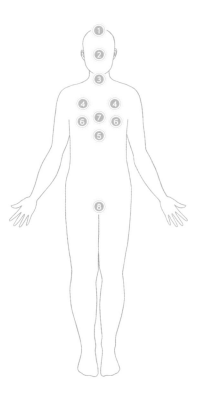

Grounding

When we can't seem to eliminate our negative, spiraling thoughts, a Reiki session for grounding may be just what the universe ordered! In addition to the treatment sequence listed here, see "Grounding Visualization Meditation" on page 170.

1. Root chakra
2. Ankles
3. Soles of the feet

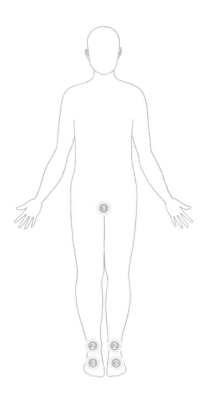

TIP: Spending more time in nature helps us feel more grounded. Walking barefoot (if possible) on the grass, dirt, and sand can help our attention return to the body and remember our connection to Earth.

AFFIRMATION

I am here, and I am safe.

GROUNDING VISUALIZATION MEDITATION

1. Sit on a chair or a place where you can plant your feet firmly on the ground.

2. Close your eyes and imagine that there are tree roots extending from the soles of your feet that connect you all the way down to the deep core of Earth.

3. When you inhale, imagine that the life force energy of Earth is traveling from the core all the way up to touch the bottom of your feet. This energy enters your body through your feet all the way to the top of your head.

4. When you exhale, your life force energy travels deep down to the core of Earth, warming Earth on its way.

5. Continue to imagine this energy exchange as you inhale and exhale, until you feel that the energy that is a part of you is also the energy that is a part of Earth.

Heartbreak

The heart doesn't physically break, but it sometimes sure feels like it! Comforting and nurturing, Reiki helps eliminate the heavy energy and clarifies the lessons this relationship brings for your evolution and growth. Invoke the Mental/Emotional Symbol (Sei Hei Ki) anytime you feel inclined throughout the treatment.

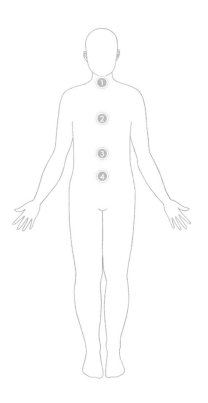

1. Throat chakra
2. Heart chakra
3. Solar plexus chakra
4. Sacral chakra

AFFIRMATION

What belongs to me will always find me.

I find love wherever I go.

Intuition

Along with a consistent meditation practice, Reiki helps one listen to and trust their inner knowing and gut feeling more confidently.

1. Crown chakra
2. Third eye chakra
3. Cupped hands placed gently over the eyes
4. Solar plexus chakra

AFFIRMATION

I am quieting my mind so I can listen to my inner voice. Everything I need is within me.

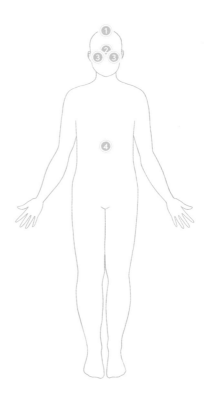

Life Purpose/Calling

When we find ourselves pondering our life calling, try focusing on what we often think about when we envision our future life. What we often think about is not random, and Reiki can help bring focus and clarity around such desires and visions.

1. Crown chakra
2. Third eye chakra
3. Throat chakra
4. Heart chakra

AFFIRMATION

Every day I am finding clues and hints
that point to my life purpose.

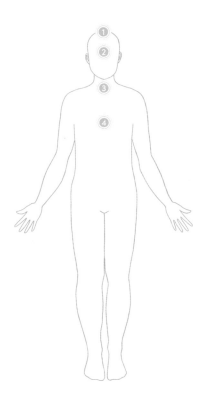

Overthinking

Overthinking is often a result of trying to resolve uncertainty about the future. Reiki helps by relieving the mind of its attachment to a specific outcome. The "Five Senses Mindfulness Exercise" on page 175 is a helpful tool to bring your focus back to the present moment.

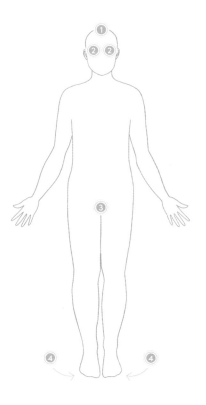

1. Crown chakra
2. Eyelids
3. Root chakra
4. Soles of the feet

AFFIRMATION

I release what I cannot control. Life is always happening for me.

FIVE SENSES MINDFULNESS EXERCISE

1. Acknowledge five things you see around you (for example, clothes, clock, water bottle, bookshelf, and windows).

2. Acknowledge four things you can touch around you (for example, bedsheets, pillow, notebook, and crystals).

3. Acknowledge three things you hear (for example, cars, television, and wind).

4. Acknowledge two things you can smell (for example, candles and fresh laundry).

5. Acknowledge one thing you can taste (for example, tea).

Security

Feeling safe and secure is a basic human need. If feelings of insecurity are an issue, during Reiki, it might be helpful for the recipient to recall their earliest childhood memory associated with feeling unsafe to explore the root of the wound. Invoke the Distant Symbol (Hon Sha Ze Sho Nen) and imagine your younger self in a gentle, protective, white bubble as you send your inner child distant Reiki. A physical self-hug lends further comfort.

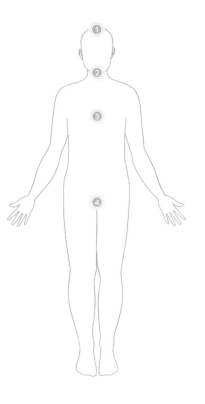

1. Crown chakra
2. Bottom of the head
3. Heart chakra
4. Root chakra

AFFIRMATION

I am safe. I feel safe. I feel the support of Earth beneath me.

Self-Esteem Issues

Reiki helps one cultivate self-acceptance and unconditional love, which can make one feel more confident by bringing the body back into a state of wholeness.

1. Top of the head
2. Back of the head
3. Forehead
4. Heart chakra
5. Solar plexus chakra

AFFIRMATION

I am stronger than my fears.

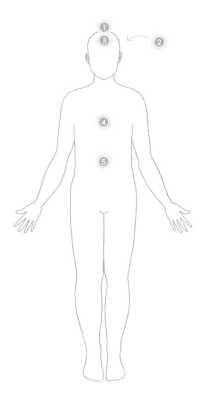

Speaking the Truth

Speaking with honesty can be quite difficult, but sometimes it is essential to change and growth. Reiki supports the need to not only stay true to who you are but to express your feelings, opinions, and morals more freely. As Reiki is being beamed to the throat, the recipient might find it helpful to make an audible "ah" sound with each exhale.

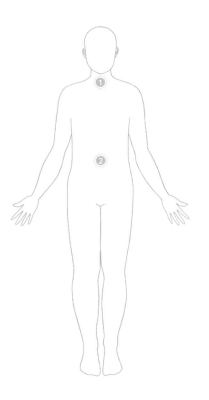

1. Throat chakra
2. Solar plexus chakra

AFFIRMATION

I speak my truth. My voice is important in this world.

Stress

When feeling stress becomes the norm rather than the exception, people find that Reiki offers a much-needed break to bring the body and mind to a state of relaxation. See also the "Visualization Meditation to Release Tension and Stress" on page 180.

1. Crown chakra
2. Cupped hands placed gently over the eyes
3. Index, middle, and ring fingers placed over eyelid with very little pressure
4. Sides of the jaw
5. Heart chakra
6. Diaphragm
7. Root chakra

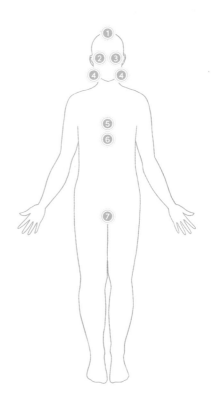

VISUALIZATION MEDITATION TO RELEASE TENSION AND STRESS

1. Come to a seated position and bring your hands to your heart center. Gently close your eyes.

2. Place your thumbs touching your heart so you can feel your heartbeat. Take a moment to tune in and listen to your breath for a while.

3. Notice every inhale, every exhale—even that moment between every inhale and exhale, that sweet spot we often miss or neglect. Inhale, widen your chest, and exhale as you ground down your energy on Earth. Inhale as you shine your heart forward to receive; exhale as you surrender your body weight to the ground supporting you.

4. Keep your eyes closed and slowly scan your body head to toe, from the crown of your head to the bottom of your feet, and determine where you are holding tension or stress in your body. There is no need to label or judge your circumstances right now. Just notice how you feel in this present moment. Notice any subtle energies or sensations you feel in your body.

5. When you find that spot in your body where you are holding tension, imagine breathing oxygen into it and around it. Imagine your bones, joints, and muscles around the area relaxing. Can you relax a little bit more? Can you let go a little bit more?

6. Draw your shoulders away from your ears, relax. Soften your fingertips, relax. Unclench your jaw, relax. And even relax your tongue. Allow your body to release tension and stress that no longer serve you.

7. You are welcome to stay here as long as you want.

Unwanted Energy

From time to time we pick up and hold on to other people's energy. We may unexplainably feel drained or somewhat ill or irritable. When this happens, we may need a cleansing of the auric field.

1. Sweep your hands from the top of the head all the way down to the bottom of the feet. Repeat three times.
2. Perform Kenyoku (see page 24).

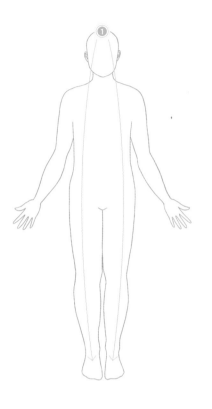

TIP: A bath with Epsom salt and Himalayan salts is a relaxing and effective way to cleanse the auric field and draw toxins from the body. I take a cleansing bath after a day of seeing clients and when I come home from a big event or if I am feeling drained. This is a pro tip for especially sensitive empaths out there like me. Alternatively, soak feet in warm/hot water mixed with the salts in a basin for about 15 minutes.

Hi there,

We hope you enjoyed reading *Reiki Illustrated*. If you have any questions or concerns about your book, or have received a damaged copy, please contact customerservice@penguinrandomhouse.com. We're here and happy to help.

Also, please consider writing a review on your favorite retailer's website to let others know what you thought of the book!

Sincerely,
The Zeitgeist Team

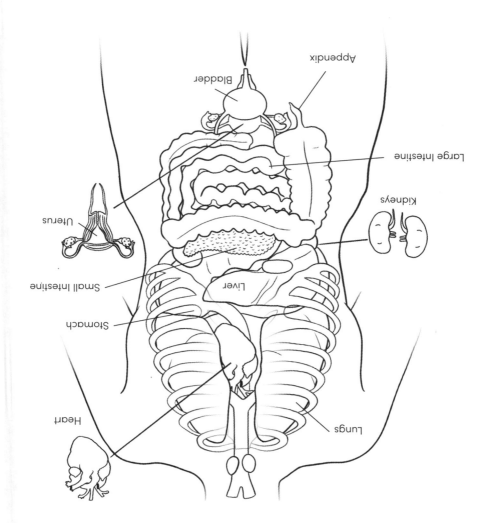

Appendix

Bladder

Large Intestine

Uterus

Kidneys

Small Intestine

Liver

Stomach

Heart

Lungs

APPENDIX

ABOUT THE AUTHOR

Hae Lee is one of the most sought-after Reiki healers and teachers in Los Angeles, California. She is passionate about helping people heal their mind, body, and spirit, as she is a firm believer that true well-being encompasses a balance and awareness of all three.

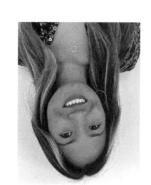

One of Hae's goals is to share and teach this beautiful healing modality—which transformed her life—with as many people as possible and prove that anyone can learn to channel Reiki to better heal and understand themselves. She has Reiki certified and trained more than 300 students from all over the world and currently teaches Reiki certification courses online. Her students find her teachings spiritual and transformative, yet very practical and grounded at the same time. Her regular clients include Hollywood producers, celebrities, and business moguls.

Hae is also currently attaining a master's degree in clinical psychology at Antioch University in hopes of creating a practice that specializes in a mind-body-spiritual approach in relation to self, others, and society. For more information, visit StayandVibe.org.

ABOUT THE ILLUSTRATOR

Natalie Foss is a Norwegian freelance illustrator and artist currently based in London. She draws primarily with colored pencils and procreate, focusing on bold colors and emotions—often portraying alienated or curious beings adorned by '60s/'70s inspired patterns and motifs. Her art is inspired by the everyday life and music. For more information, visit nataliefoss.co.uk or follow her on Instagram @nat.foss.

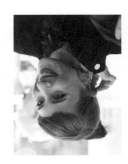

INDEX

Page numbers in *italics* indicate illustrations.